MANAGEMENT of SWALLOWING and TUBE FEEDING in ADULTS:

A TEAM APPROACH

ANITA RUSSELL *SPEECH PATHOLOGIST*
& PETER HILL *DIETITIAN*

with a Foreword by **MICHAEL E. GROHER Ph. D.**

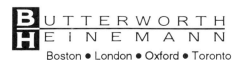

BUTTERWORTH
HEINEMANN
Boston • London • Oxford • Toronto

7-98

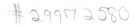

MANAGEMENT OF SWALLOWING AND TUBE FEEDING IN ADULTS
is the international edition of
TRANSITIONAL FEEDING, Second Edition,
which was printed and published in Australia.

ISBN 0-7506-9560-9

Production and Printing: AL Printers
Original Publisher: JF Foundation P.O. Box 221 Unley S.A. 5061 Australia
Distributed by: Butterworth-Heinemann
80 Montvale Avenue, Stoneham. MA 02180 U.S.A.

CONTENTS

FOREWORD

For the past decade, a considerable amount of attention has been given to the care of patients with oropharyngeal dysphagia.

It is clear that the most successful outcomes of this care result from the co-operative efforts of many specialists, particularly speech-language pathologists, nurses, dietitians, and attending physicians.

Co-ordinating these efforts is a difficult task, which is why this practical reference, written by two experienced and skilled professionals is such a welcome addition to the literature.

For team members involved in the care of adults with acquired neurological deficit, *Management of Swallowing and Tube Feeding in Adults* will serve as an effective and useful guide.

It is a concise, well-organized reference for solving the diagnostic and treatment dilemmas of patients at every level of alimentation, from tube feeding decisions to early attempts at oral ingestion, to moving from a soft to a regular diet. Throughout it conveys to the reader the need to consider each aspect of a patient's diagnosis, history, and present medical status before formulating a treatment plan.

Beginning clinicians will appreciate the book's explicit detail and firm direction. Advanced clinicians will find it to be a useful resource, and they will use it to improve the development of the multidisciplinary team approach in dysphagia management.

Finally, this manual conveys the expert knowledge of its authors, a speech pathologist and a dietitian. Only clinicians with considerable experience in the trenches could have achieved such a perfect combination of clinical direction and clinical intuition. Their presentation will be of considerable value to all involved in the management of those with oropharyngeal dysphagia and its secondary manifestations.

Michael E. Groher, Ph. D.
James A. Haley Veterans Hospital
Tampa, Florida

November, 1993

PREFACE

Julia Farr Centre, located in Adelaide in the Australian State of South Australia, is an organisation which provides a wide range of rehabilitation services. It has provided services to people with physical disabilities since 1878, but many of the Allied Health Disciplines have only been introduced over the last ten years, co-inciding with an increased emphasis on rehabilitation.

Julia Farr Centre has a large residential component comprising three main elements:

- A long-term care component of approximately 350 people with a variety of neurological conditions, either congenital or acquired.
  Medical diagnoses within this group include Multiple Sclerosis, Motor Neurone Disease, Huntington's Disease, Advanced Parkinson's Disease, Stroke, and congenital neurological disorders such as cerebral palsy.
  There is also an increasing number of people who have survived very severe head injuries.

- A rehabilitation/convalescence service of approx. 40 beds, which admits people discharged from acute hospitals for short-term rehabilitation.

- The South Australian Head Injury Service (approx. 20 beds) conducting fast stream rehabilitation leading to discharge into the community. The Head Injury Service also conducts an outpatient service and a community integration service.

As each of these new services has been added, the range of Allied Health Disciplines has increased, as well as the numbers of professionals in each of these disciplines. New treatments and techniques have been adopted as standard practice; and assessment, monitoring and evaluation techniques have also evolved.

This book describes procedures which have been developed over time at the Julia Farr Centre, when treating people suffering from dysphagia.

It is evident the involvement of a team of professionals, as well as carers, is very important. The speech pathologist and the dietitian obviously play key roles in this process, and people from these disciplines have combined to write this book, which we hope will assist many people receiving care in a wide range of situations.

Humphry A. McGrath
President and Chairman, Board of Directors.
Julia Farr Centre.

About the authors:

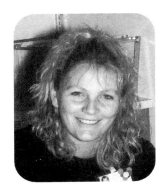

Anita Russell is a Speech Pathologist who was employed at Julia Farr Centre. at the time of writing this book

Awarded a Queen Elizabeth II Silver Jubilee Scholarship, Anita travelled to the U.S.A and to the U.K. under the award, and during this time she obtained valuable additional experience through discussions with practioners pre-eminent in the field of dysphagia.

On her return to South Australia, she introduced many new ideas into the development of this book.

Anita is at present living in Singapore and working as Director of Clinical Services at the Tan Sen Hok Hospital.

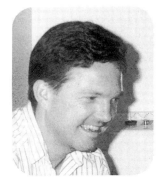

Peter Hill is a Senior Dietitian who worked at Julia Farr Centre during the writing of this book.

He had worked assiduously to improve the diets and nutrition at the Julia Farr Centre, and has continued his interest by updating the dietary information in this edition.

Peter, for some time, conducted a part-time private practice in Nutrition, with professional advice to nursing homes and hospitals. He was frequently in demand to provide staff development in organisations throughout Australia, and helped with the production of an instructional video entitled "The Enteral Connection" for a commercial organisation.

Peter at present lives and works in the U.K.

ACKNOWLEDGEMENTS

We are fortunate to have worked at Julia Farr Centre at a time when such rapid development of services was taking place. The Centre's philosophy of care required ongoing improvement to services, the recognition of the rights of clients and their carers and the establishment of outcome standards.

We wish to thank our allied health, medical, nursing and catering colleagues at Julia Farr Centre who are committed to the processes of providing client care through a multidisciplinary team approach. Their encouragement and willingness to accept change has been a source of inspiration.

The authors are especially indebted to Julia Farr Foundation Incorporated for funding the production of this manual and accompanying training video. We gratefully acknowledge their ongoing commitment to research and development in the care of clients with disability.

The authors would also like to thank Butterworth/Heinemann, for their advice and assistance in converting the Australian Text to an international edition.

Anita Russell
and Peter Hill

INTRODUCTION

'Transitional Feeding - The Team Approach' clinical manual and video has been successfully received world-wide by health professionals, training schools, volunteer organisations and family carers. Our new revised edition is in response to numerous requests to expand detail in the areas of assessment and intervention. Newly devised checklists, flowcharts and standards of intervention are intended to promote quality assurance in practice. Finally the recognition and discussion of variations in professional opinion and therapeutic practice will ensure that this comprehensive resource is valid now and in the future.

At Julia Farr Centre we have had extensive experience with clients who present with acquired neurological swallowing deficits.

Some have progressive and inexorably fatal neurological conditions, particularly motor neurone disease (amyotrophic lateral sclerosis). The aim with them is to provide support and to maintain safe care in a terminal illness.

Others have suffered trauma or disease, with an expectation of improvement and varying degrees of recovery. Often they (or more often their families) are keen to start feeding too soon. They need careful evaluation and the support of experienced staff while progressing through transitional feeding.

In both of these situations a client undergoing transitional feeding is in a potentially hazardous situation, from aspiration with respiratory complications, and from the sequelae of inadequate nutrition and hydration. Those who feed these dependent people, and the clients themselves, face great frustration and sometimes anxiety. Feeding seems such a natural function that it is hard for some people to accept that expert help from a multidisciplinary team is required. Staff who have had bad experiences can be apprehensive at the prospect of embarking on a transitional feeding program, with unfortunate implications for the client.

We heavily emphasise the great contribution by family members. We see them as being very much full members of the therapeutic team, and adequate time must be taken to educate and support them. We have repeatedly found that the personality of the feeder is more important than professional or educational status, and management must be sufficiently flexible to accept this.

The aims of our programs and procedures are to achieve the highest potential for the client to enjoy a normal life of high quality.

Any disruption in the initiation, co-ordination and maintenance of a swallow through weakness, delay or paralysis, can give rise to the clinical condition known as dysphagia. The cause, degree of impairment and prognosis are determined by the speech pathologist and medical officer.

All team members are committed to the philosophies of:

1. Objective and comprehensive assessment of a client's strengths and deficits.

2. Prevention of undue physical and emotional stress.

3. Continuing evaluation and review.

4. Employing skilled observation and standardised assessments.

5. Education and information sharing amongst all caregivers, including family members.

Involvement of specific health disciplines will depend largely on the composition of the team and the evolving needs of the client.

Early referral and assessment are most useful in estimating the likely time for recovery or deterioration. In our experience the swallowing process can not be successfully assessed or treated if approached in isolation from the rest of the person. Different team members will provide specific expertise and come together to establish a baseline of function, to plan priorities, and to implement and review short and long term goals in management.

The aims of transitional feeding are:

1. The safe and adequate intake of nutrition, hydration and medication.

2. Maximum quality of life, including independence, variety, time and self-esteem.

3. Prevention of further complications in overall nutrition and medical status.

There is no precise time schedule for transitional feeding programs, because outcome can be affected by many human and physical variables. Ideally, wherever a multidisciplinary team exists in a rehabilitation or palliative care facility, transitional feeding can be undertaken - for example in acute hospitals, long-stay institutions, hospices and rehabilitation centres. Acute and long-term facilities will undoubtedly vary in their emphasis on overall management as the needs of clients change with their medical conditions.

Whether it is the transition from eating to alternative feeding, or from alternative feeding to eating, the goal is to improve wellness and achieve a level of eating or feeding satisfactory to the wishes of the client and caregivers.

It will be seen that we distinguish between eating, which is the process in which a person can personally place food and drink in the mouth before a swallow, and feeding, when another person has to do that, or when alternative methods must be used, usually by tube.

ON CLIENTS, DIGRAPHS, SIGNIFICANT OTHERS, AND MEDICAL OFFICERS

All of our efforts are directed to the person who needs help with eating, who is described as the `client` rather than as the `patient`.

Since January 1988 Julia Farr Centre has followed the spelling convention of the World Health Organization. Generally speaking this follows American usage, so we write `esophagus`, not `oesophagus`.

We describe those concerned for the welfare of the client as `family` or family members. We accept that they may not be formally related by blood or marriage, but we wish to avoid jargon terms such as `significant other`.

The term medical officer describes any suitably trained medical physician.

Anita Russell
Peter Hill

1

ASSESSMENT - AN OVERVIEW

Assessment of swallowing, eating and/or feeding difficulties provides a blueprint for therapy. Observation, direct assessment, and trials of treatment strategies are all utilised to provide comprehensive information regarding the client's 'swallowing system'.

Symptoms or warning signs of a disorder in either swallowing, eating or feeding may have a variety of origins. Physical symptoms may include coughing, choking, drooling, pocketing of food, or weight loss and dehydration. Emotional indicators may appear as a fear of eating, avoidance of food types, depression or fatigue. Feeder factors commonly include uncertainty or fear regarding emergency procedures, non-compliance with prescribed food/fluid recommendations, poor documentation and changes in skill level with alterations in staffing levels.

Therefore to assume that a simple assessment of the gag reflex or lip and tongue muscles will determine the best possible management of swallowing, eating or feeding difficulties is indeed naive.

An interdisciplinary team of trained health professionals is needed to investigate the swallowing system.

Therapists responsible for the assessment of swallowing disorders should consult Logemann[1] and Groher[2] for a thorough explanation of the anatomy and physiology of normal swallow and the various pathologies giving rise to the condition known as dysphagia.

In this manual we will concentrate on swallowing, eating and feeding difficulties as a direct result of acquired neurological conditions, i.e.

> traumatic-head injury, cerebro-vascular accident,
> hypoxia, tumour progressive-dementia, idiopathic,
> inherited infectious-meningitis

On receipt of a referral the swallowing team, comprising key health professionals and family carers, may commence a comprehensive assessment of the swallowing system. The assessment process is not haphazard. Instead it consists of three sequential steps:

1. **Before Eating Assessment Flowchart** is used as an initial guide to establishing baseline functions. It alerts each team member to make an observation of the various factors that may invariably affect swallowing, eating or feeding ability. Information obtained can determine the appropriateness of a referral and the need for further detailed assessment. Strengths and issues are highlighted.

2. **Direct Assessment of Swallow** requires a skilled health professional to investigate the competency of the oral, velo-pharyngeal, pharyngeal

BEFORE EATING ASSESSMENT FLOWCHART

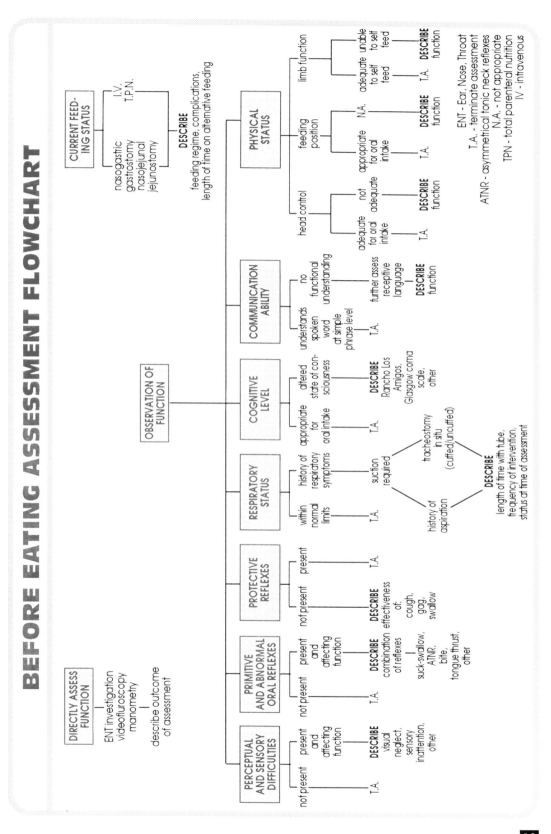

DIRECTLY ASSESS FUNCTION
- ENT investigation
- videofluroscopy
- manometry
- describe outcome of assessment

CURRENT FEEDING STATUS
- nasogastric
- gastrostomy
- nasojejunal
- jejunostomy
- I.V.
- T.P.N.

DESCRIBE
feeding regime, complications, length of time on alternative feeding

OBSERVATION OF FUNCTION

PERCEPTUAL AND SENSORY DIFFICULTIES
- not present → T.A.
- present and affecting function → **DESCRIBE** visual neglect, sensory inattention, other

PRIMITIVE AND ABNORMAL ORAL REFLEXES
- not present → T.A.
- present and affecting function → **DESCRIBE** combination of reflexes i.e. suck-swallow, ATNR, bite, tongue thrust, other

PROTECTIVE REFLEXES
- present → T.A.
- not present → **DESCRIBE** effectiveness of: cough, gag, swallow

RESPIRATORY STATUS
- within normal limits → T.A.
- history of respiratory symptoms
- suction required
- tracheostomy in situ (cuffed/uncuffed)
- history of aspiration

DESCRIBE length of time with tube, frequency of intervention, status at time of assessment

COGNITIVE LEVEL
- appropriate for oral intake → T.A.
- altered state of consciousness → **DESCRIBE** Rancho Los Amigos, Glasgow coma scale, other

COMMUNICATION ABILITY
- understands spoken word at simple phrase level → T.A.
- no functional understanding → further assess receptive language i.e. **DESCRIBE** function

PHYSICAL STATUS

head control
- adequate for oral intake → T.A.
- not adequate → **DESCRIBE** function

feeding position
- appropriate for oral intake → T.A.
- N.A. → **DESCRIBE** function

limb function
- adequate to self feed
- unable to self feed → T.A. → **DESCRIBE** function

ENT - Ear, Nose, Throat
T.A. - terminate assessment
ATNR - asymmetrical tonic neck reflexes
N.A. - not appropriate
TPN - total parenteral nutrition
IV - intravenous

ASSESSMENT OF THE SWALLOWING SYSTEM

Medical Factors
- Diagnosis
- Prognosis
- Surgical, pharmacological management
- Stability
- Co-existing medical conditions

Emotional Factors
- Fear of choking
- Mourning lost functions
- Depression

Ethical Factors
- Informed consent
- Testamentary capacity
- Duty of care
- Beneficence
- Non-maleficence
- Rights

Family Carers
- Understanding & expectations
- Level of involvement
- Advisory role
- Advocacy role
- Infantalism

Physical Factors
- Motor and sensory function of oral, pharyngeal and esophageal phases of swallow
- Nutritional requirements
- Respiratory system functions
- Body and head positioning
- Level of independence

Feeder Factors
- Skill level
- Support and supervision
- Paternalism
- Fear of choking
- Resistance to change

Communication Factors
- Functional understanding
- Functional expression

Cognitive Factors
- Behaviour and judgement
- New learning
- Awareness

EATING • FEEDING • SWALLOWING

CLIENT

and esophageal stage of swallow. The adequacy of the protective reflexes (cough, gag, swallow) determine safety for oral intake. Various treatment techniques may be utilized and their effects noted. Strengths and issues are highlighted and potential for improvement with treatment is estimated.

Radiographic investigation through video fluroscopy, and manometry testing may be useful in identifying precisely what has gone wrong in the velo-pharyngeal, pharyngeal, and esophogeal stage of swallow.

Note:
> Video fluroscopy requires advanced preparation, time and a strong hypothesis regarding probable cause(s) and treatment options in order to maximise the meaning of results obtained for future management.

3. **Eating Assessment Flowchart** assists the team in compiling relevant information and determining the level at which the client is best and safest with various textures and consistencies. Initial decisions are made regarding treatment priorities in the Before Eating and Eating areas.

After assessments are completed the intervention process begins. A detailed account of swallowing, eating and feeding management forms the basis of this manual.

EATING ASSESSMENT FLOWCHART

SALIVA
- manages own saliva → T.A.
- has difficulties swallowing own saliva

FREE FLUIDS
- manages free fluids with no difficulties → T.A.
- does not manage free fluids

VITAMISED DIET
- manages this texture with no difficulties → T.A.
- does not manage vitamised texture

MINCED DIET
- manages this texture with no difficulties → T.A.
- does not manage minced texture

SOLIDS
- manages this texture with no difficulties → T.A.
- does not manage solids

FURTHER ASSESS

COGNITIVE DIFFICULTIES
- not contributing to swallowing function → T.A.
- present and affecting swallowing function
  - **DESCRIBE** initiation, awareness, orientation, memory

PHYSICAL STATUS
- no difficulties → T.A.
- demonstrates physical difficulty contributing to swallow dysfunction
  - assess oral stage
    - **DESCRIBE** dysarthria, swallow reflex, dental problems, compensatory techniques
  - assess velo-pharyngeal stage
    - **DESCRIBE** nasal regurgitation, swallow reflex - (delay/absent) posterior tongue movement
  - assess pharyngeal stage
    - **DESCRIBE** protective reflexes, swallow reflex, transit time, motility, reflux, other
  - assess esophageal stage
    - **DESCRIBE** reflux, vomiting, regurgitation

DESCRIBE OVERALL LEVEL OF FUNCTION
- adequate
- adequate but reduced
- non-functional

MODIFICATIONS TO TEXTURE
- none required → T.A.
- modifications present
  - **DESCRIBE** thickeners, bamix, other

NUTRITIONAL HISTORY
- uneventful → T.A.
- demonstrates nutritional problems
  - **DESCRIBE** malnutrition, dehydration, weight loss, food preferences, other

T.A. - terminate assessment

16

A GUIDE to the ASSESSMENT of DYSPHAGIA

Referral and Case Records

- Review medical records and extrapolate relevant information regarding location and extent of cortical lesion (s).
- Note provisional diagnosis and guarded prognosis. List other concurrent medical conditions which may effect future swallow management.
- Note results of cranial nerve testing (v, vii, ix, x, xii) and any previous direct or indirect swallow investigations (see chapter 6).
- Note any previous swallowing management, including surgical intervention, unorthodox treatments (in both the institution and community).
- Note relevant communications between therapists and consultants regarding tempo of recovery / decline, carer support system, client motivation, insight judgement, and fatigue.

Cognitive and Communication Ability

- Note relevant coma scales (Glasgow Coma Scale) and functioning on outcome scales (Rancho Los Amigo Scale - see page 133).
- Note effectiveness of verbal and non-verbal communication using informal assessment or formal testing at appropriate level. (eg. Western Neurological Sensory Stimulation Profile, Frenchay Dysarthria Assessment.)
- Note client awareness, insight, motivation and wishes regarding swallowing status and management.

Direct Assessment of Swallow

- *Reflexive Examination:* Undertake assessment of Gag, Cough and Swallow Reflex.
- *Preparatory Phase Examination:* Note perceptual and sensory difficulties, initiation and distractability. (See Before Eating Flowchart).
- *Oral Phase Examination:* Undertake assessment of the muscles of the face, mouth and tongue (eg. Eating Flowchart, Frenchay Dysarthria Profile, Rehabilitation Institute of Chicago - Swallowing Assessment) and note presence and effect of oral reflexes; abnormal muscle tone; abnormal sensation; movement disorders and dental and oral hygiene.
- *Pharyngeal Phase Examination:* Undertake assessment of swallow efficiency and the likelihood of aspiration ie: history of aspiration; spontaneous and facilitated swallow (feeling the larynx, stethoscope to hear swallow); phonation test. Note: Further radiographic investigation using videofluroscopy may be indicated for clients demonstrating ++ aspiration and the possibility of significant pharyngeal phase dysfunction.
- *Esophageal Phase Examination:* If reflux and resultant aspiration is noted, further radiological and manometry investigation of the cricopharyngeal / gastro-esophageal sphincter is required.

Summarise Data and make Recommendations

- Compile information from "Before Eating" and "Eating" Flowcharts with that obtained from Direct Bedside Assessment.
- Recommend readiness for oral intake, need for alternative feeding, and /or supplements, including mode of delivery for medication.
- Ensure assessment findings and team decisions regarding swallow management (including Key team members) are clearly documented in case records and relevant 'other' working documents. ie: Nursing Care Plan.

CHAPTER 1 REFERENCES
Assessment - an overview

1. Logemann J. *Evaluation and treatment of swallowing disorders*. San Diego: College-Hill Press Inc., 1983.
2. Groher ME (ed) *Dysphagia: diagnosis and management*. Boston: Butterworths, 1984.

2

TRANSITION FROM EATING TO ALTERNATIVE FEEDING

Swallowing dysfunction associated with degenerative neurological disease, such as motor neurone disease, is progressive and irreversible. [1,2,3,4]

Primary assessments establish an individual's ability to maintain eating and determine the need for introduction of alternative feeding before there is an acute clinical crisis.

Intervention is aimed at maximising residual function, anticipating future decline in swallowing, and presenting clients with alternative feeding options should eating become too difficult: namely naso-gastric, gastrostomy or jejunostomy tube feeding. The timing and degree of intervention are determined in consultation with the client, family and staff.

Introduction of alternative feeding before a predictable crisis has many advantages in the maintenance of quality of life, for example rehydration, adequate pain relief and reduced anxiety. [2,5] Some clients will choose to continue normal eating for much longer than is advised or may be safe, and in reality may change preference for alternative feeding versus normal eating a number of times as the disease progresses. Although professional caregivers have an obligation to present all management options, the client is under no obligation to comply with any one of these.

The matter of safety in such a situation can cause great and justifiable anxiety to all caregivers.

Ethically our obligation is primarily to the client, not to those who may be profoundly concerned for the welfare of the client, whether they be members of the family or professionals.

If a rational client with full legal and testamentary capacity makes an informed and consistent decision to continue or to abandon treatment all involved are bound by that decision and must act accordingly.

In this chapter a description of the general principles and procedures is followed by specific strategies for management of swallowing in the advanced phase of specific diseases, namely motor neurone disease, Huntington's disease, Parkinson's disease and multiple sclerosis.

Involvement of individual members of the supporting team will largely depend on the composition of the team and the evolving needs of the client. Commonly the ideal professional team may not exist under one roof, so an appropriate referral may be required to seek out particular expertise from another agency.

FAMILY

Provides information on the client's cultural background, lifestyle and food preferences. Participation in programs is welcomed, and family members are encouraged to evaluate and review progress, and to suggest changes.

SPEECH PATHOLOGIST

Offers direct assessment, diagnosis and treatment of impaired swallowing and eating ability, and participates in education, liaison, review processes and generally co-ordinates the team.

DIETITIAN

Undertakes assessment of current and past nutritional status and also determines future nutritional requirements. Translates nutritional requirements into appropriate foods, fluids and formulae. Advises on tube feeding regimes.

MEDICAL OFFICER

Monitors ongoing medical status, advises on the impact of medical conditions on swallowing, and may prescribe medications, further investigations or surgical procedures.

NURSE

Monitors and implements the prescribed feeding program and assesses, reviews and reports progress to team members to evaluate change.

PHYSIOTHERAPIST

Offers assessment of respiratory status, including the effectiveness of protective cough reflex, oro-pharyngeal suctioning requirements, as well as advising on total body posture and positioning for feeding: for example, head control or chair position.

OCCUPATIONAL THERAPIST

Assesses correct posture and level of independence in feeding, and also determines the need for therapeutic aids for eating and feeding.

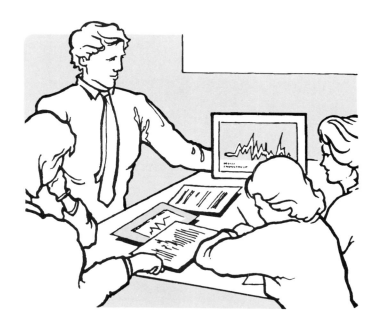

SOCIAL WORKER

Undertakes an assessment of the client's immediate support system and ensures that the individual's rights are upheld. Provides liaison and support to all caregivers (family and professionals).

DENTIST

Provides overall assessment of dental status, including oral hygiene, dentures and swallowing prosthesis where appropriate. Preventive dentistry is encouraged.

Note:
Roles of individual team members may differ between institutions, home-care facilities, different states and countries. Often roles will merge depending on the emphasis of the service and individual skills and experiences of team members.

EVALUATION

Procedures and flowcharts used in the assessment process are summarised in Chapters 1 and 4 of this manual.

The evaluation process (in terms of both process and outcome) should begin as soon after referral as possible. Information is obtained from a variety of objective, standardised and non-standardised assessments through direct observation, and by undertaking a detailed case history. [6]

There are six main areas to be evaluated and information should be obtained regarding each of the following:

1. Medical condition.
2. Eating and swallowing ability.
3. Nutritional status.
4. Physical status.
5. Level of independence.
6. Emotional state.

1. MEDICAL CONDITION

Evaluation of a client's medical condition incorporates: [6,7,8]

1.1 A description of the present illness, including signs and symptoms, onset and character, and any treatments, factors or behaviours that aggravate or improve symptoms.

1.2 The client and caregivers' descriptions of the present medical condition, with emphasis on any co-existing illnesses and treatment.

1.3 A thorough neurological examination of higher cortical functions, motor and sensory systems and normal/abnormal reflex pathways is aimed at confirming the presence and tempo of progressive disease. Physical examination is commonly accompanied by neurodiagnostic, imaging and biochemical evaluation.

1.4 A review of orthodox professional, and unorthodox or alternative services, diets and medications sought during the course of the illness.

1.5 Confirmation that all involved have a good understanding of the nature and implications of the disease or injury, with the natural history and prognosis.

2. EATING AND SWALLOWING ABILITY

Adequacy in eating and swallowing is evaluated by a speech pathologist. A detailed examination consists of making assessments of the client's competence with food and fluids in each of the swallowing phases:

2.1 ORAL PHASE [9,10,11]

- Lips —
  Closure of the lips seals the oral cavity. Food or fluid may leak from the mouth, causing drooling which may embarrass the client.

- Jaw —
  Movements of the mandible produce a chewing action. The ability to manipulate, form, hold and propel food posteriorly may be reduced. Ill-fitting dentures may compound chewing difficulties.

- Tongue —
  Food is moved by the tongue between the teeth for chewing and backward toward the pharynx to facilitate initiation of the swallowing reflex. Weakness and/or reduced sensation can result in food or fluids falling into the cheek sulcus or escaping over the base of the tongue before a swallow reflex is stimulated. This is shown by aspiration (entry of particles into the airway) before the swallow. (see page 119)

- Face—
  Movements of the cheek and surrounding lip muscles hold food in contact with the teeth. As a result of food pocketing in the cheek, gum disease, caries and bad breath may result.

2.2 VELOPHARYNGEAL PHASE [9,11,12]

- Soft Palate—
  Contractions of a number of muscles in and around the soft palate close off the nasal passages from the pharynx. Food and fluid may be regurgitated through the nose if weakness or paralysis is evidenced by a diminished or absent gag reflex.

- Protective Reflexes—
  A detailed description of the cough and swallow reflex is noted spontaneously and on command. Aspiration and choking may occur if there is absent or diminished function.

2.3 PHARYNGEAL PHASE [3,4,13,14]

- Laryngeal musculature—
  Excursion of the larynx forward and upward assists in closing off the

airway. Weakness, paralysis or inco-ordination in this phase can result in airway obstruction during or after the swallow.

- Cricopharyngeal muscle—
  Food and fluid is passed into the upper esophagus by relaxation of this sphincter. Spasm and inco-ordination can result in overflow into the airway, resulting in aspiration after the swallow.

3. NUTRITIONAL STATUS

Current nutritional status is evaluated by a dietitian who determines the client's optimal nutritional needs. This involves examination of all factors that can affect a person's requirements and subsequent intake. Nutrition intervention strategies can then be agreed upon in conjunction with the client and family.[12,15]

3.1 DIET HISTORY

The diet history is taken on admission and provides a qualitative and quantitative picture of the client's food behaviour patterns and consumption.

Information usually obtained will include:

Help available at home for purchasing and preparing meals and labour saving equipment, such as food processors or blenders, will give an idea of how much effort will be available and required for meal preparation.

Modification techniques used by the client or caregivers in preparing meals, are encouraged where appropriate as these have been accepted by the client.

General food preferences e.g. savoury, sweet, spicy etc., including foods that are currently enjoyed, easily eaten foods and foods that are excluded due to taste change, difficulty in chewing or for safety reasons. Current use of commercial foods or supplements is also noted.

Food beliefs held by the client or family should be respected and alternative choices found if there is potential for nutritional compromise, e.g. non-dairy products, vegetarian diets etc. If the client is ambivalent about his or her beliefs and shows an open attitude for change, scientific evidence should be made available, so the client may make an informed decision.

Weight history including usual weight, height to calculate health weight, estimated ideal weight, and rate of weight change.

Record of a typical day (24 hours) food and fluid intake, estimating amount consumed and variations in eating patterns. Observe signs of clinical malnutrition such as dehydration, constipation, rapid weight loss etc.

Food frequency and variety of foods usually eaten and identification of inadequacies from major food groups.Foods difficult to chew such as cereal foods and meat may be avoided as these often require modification.

Timing and frequency of intake of foods and fluids. This may vary depending on usual eating habits, fitting in with family commitments, convenience or fatigue.

3.2 ADEQUACY ASSESSMENT

The client's pre-admission food intake is assessed for adequacy to meet the client's nutritional needs. *Usually this will involve:*

Nutritional assessment of a 24 hour intake or food intake chart to identify specific nutrient intake and inadequacies, along with usual food intake, preferences, eating times etc.

Determining nutrient requirements from medical examination, recommended daily intakes, body stores and nutrient utilisation.

Weekly weigh to achieve and maintain ideal weight as determined by calculated ideal weight, weight history and discussion with client.

3.3 INTERVENTION

Planned intervention in the form of a nutritional care plan is offered to assist the client in planning food intake either at home or in the institutional setting.

A food plan should:

Translate specific nutrient requirements into quantities of safe and preferred foods. In conjunction with the client and family compile a meal plan or typical day's menu.

Recommend food items with or without modifications based on diet history. Suggest modifications to existing recipes or offer suitable new recipes.

Offer oral supplements with instructions on cost, availability, usual preparation techniques and use in combination with foods.

3.4 ASSESS INTERVENTION ADEQUACY

It is essential for the Dietitian to:

Re-evaluate the effectiveness and acceptance of suggested foods and modifications. In doing so he/she must consider the desires of the client to eat the volume and types of foods required to meet nutritional goals.

3.5 ALTERNATIVES

The Dietitian may suggest alternatives to oral intake such as:

1. To offer and trial the use of nutrient dense, small volume dietary supplements to reduce or replace the need to eat large volumes of food.

   or

2. Where recreational foods and drinks are eaten by the client as desired with predominant nutrition and hydration from tube feeding.

A pre-implementation evaluation will determine:

- Mode of monitoring procedures. It is imperative that staff should be trained to chart and identify adequate feeding intake, fluid balance, weight and tolerance such as regular aspiration of stomach contents, abdominal distension or gut pain after feed, reflux or heart burn and dumping syndrome.

- Tube location, which is generally into the stomach except where reflux aspiration or altered stomach emptying is present and small intestine feeding is preferable.

- Tube type as determined by anticipated duration of tube feeding.

- Formulae and fluid requirements are dependent on medical condition and gut function e.g. polymeric or elemental formulae, fluid restriction etc.

- Feeding regime aims to allow maximum independence and "feed free" times for client quality of life.

- Anticipating complications avoids undue stress to the client.

4. PHYSICAL STATUS

Examination of physical status is conducted by direct evaluation of each of the following areas:

4.1 RESPIRATORY

(See Aspiration, Choking and Emergency Procedures, Chapter 5)

- Expansion and auscultation to determine air entry.

- Cough and sputum.

- Vitalograph and peakflow measurements.

- Radiological studies, including cine or video contrast investigations.

Progressive deterioration in swallowing can significantly increase the likelihood of aspiration and repeated bouts of infection, including aspiration pneumonia. [4,12,15] When the ability to cough becomes ineffective and unproductive the need for oral/pharyngeal suction is determined.

4.2 LIMB, TRUNK AND HEAD CONTROL

Body posture is obviously important, and relevant factors include: [10,11,17]

- Sensation, joint position sense.

- Tone, contractures.

- Co-ordination in limbs and trunk.

- Active motor function.

- Range of movement.

- Sitting balance (dynamic and static).

- Wheelchair needs.

Overall degeneration in the medical condition will result in progressive loss of motor ability for feeding.

Attention to head control and posture for eating, both independently and assisted, are examined.

5. LEVEL OF INDEPENDENCE

Evaluation of independence in feeding involves direct examination of the following areas:

5.1 POSITIONING [11,18]

- Head, arm and hand in relation to food and drink.

- Functional upper limb movements for self-feeding.

- Furniture in dining area, e.g. wheelchair at table; tray on wheelchair; overbed table in bed.

- Effect of visual inattention, visual field deficit or neglect of part of the body image.

5.2 PREPARATION AND FEEDING [2,10]

- Cultural significance and implications of food preferences and eating habits are crucial factors.

- Reactive depression, fear of eating, discomfort and distress, prolonged feeding time and altered appetite may all affect mealtime behaviour and attitudes.

- Tableware, including suitable cutlery and crockery, should be carefully considered.

- Independence and reliability in meal selection and preparation should be supported as long as possible.

- Awareness and level of distractibility must be assessed.

- Use of protective garments such as a towelling apron, should be considered with due regard to the effect on self-esteem for the client and visitors.

- Splinting, weighted cuffs, and a winged head rest may be helpful.

- Fatigue and motivation are key factors, which often fluctuate during the course of the illness.

Eating and drinking are significant social aspects of most cultures, so the progressive loss of normal ability and food choices may cause embarrassment and acute stress to clients and their families.

6. EMOTIONAL STATUS

Evaluation of a client's emotional status and reaction to progressive and relentless loss of independence require careful assessment in the following areas:

6.1 ADJUSTMENT TO PROGRESSIVE DISEASE

For example, the grief process and level of acceptance and understanding of imminent changes in lifestyle.

6.2 COPING STRATEGIES

For example, specific caregiver involvement and anticipation of future decline; level of support and respite.

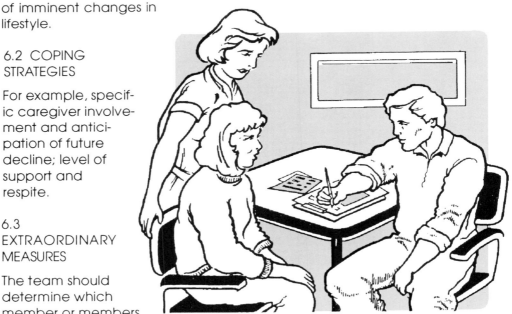

6.3 EXTRAORDINARY MEASURES

The team should determine which member or members

will undertake discussion about the option of aggressive versus non-aggressive treatment. Clients should receive sensitive support in coming to a decision on the use of artificial means to maintain nutrition and ventilation. Such important decisions are validated with family members.

The South Australian Natural Death Act provides an option to specify an explicit direction on not to use 'extraordinary measures' to prolong life in the face of progressive and inevitably fatal disease.

For the legally competent client the main intent of the 'Natural Death Act' (1983) [31] is:

- to relieve the family and health professionals of the responsibility of deciding on the nature of treatment for a client who is terminally ill and unconscious.

- to allow the formerly competent client's wishes to be respected and upheld.

- to remove the fear that clients will be subjected to the use of artificial life support during the last stages of a terminal disease.

- to allow the client to specify which procedures he or she considers as extraordinary, e.g. tube feeding.

Such decisions (which in this situation may often not be final and irrevocable) should be clearly recorded and made known to all concerned with ongoing management, including those who may be only occasionally involved.

The authors believe the "Natural Death Act" is unique to the State of South Australia, Australia. We recommend that professional staff in other states and countries investigate the existence of similar legislation and ensure that they are familiar with its principles and limitations.

DETERIORATING FUNCTION

☑ *IRREVERSIBLE SWALLOWING DYSFUNCTION*
- Maintenance therapy and compensatory techniques are not maintaining function at a safe level by oral intake.

☑ *INABILITY TO MAINTAIN DAILY REQUIREMENTS FOR FOOD AND FLUIDS*
- Malnutrition and dehydration are present or imminent.
- Consequential secondary problems arise, such as hyper-natremia and uremia.

☑ *ADMINISTRATION OF MEDICATIONS CANNOT BE MAINTAINED BY ORAL MEANS*
- Sedation and pain relief.
- Essential drugs to maintain life cannot be given comfortably by mouth.

☑ *QUALITY OF LIFE*
- The client asks for relief from hunger and thirst.
- The client's wish to continue a life regarded as active and satisfying.

THIS SECTION REFERS TO CLIENTS FACING A TERMINAL ILLNESS

Intervention in progressive disease is aimed at maintaining independence in eating and feeding for as long as it is safe and practicable.[11] The goal of this form of transitional feeding is a gradual transition from eating orally to alternative feeding as the main source of nutrition and hydration.

A clear, objective description of the client's presenting strengths and issues or areas of difficulty is essential in planning management strategies.

1. STRENGTHS

Client strengths refer to assessed areas of ability that can be utilised in transitional feeding with positive effect or outcome.

For example:

- The ability to make informed decisions about future management, which ideally should be consistent, obviously helps all concerned.

- Early intervention helps to increase awareness and facilitates acceptance by the client and family of the implications of the clinical situation.

- The client should be encouraged to accept a trial period of aids and devices to promote maximum independence.

- Discuss alternative or unorthodox treatments which may be used to alleviate specific symptoms, to help all involved to confront their emotional responses to the situation.

- Effective and functional communication of needs and wishes must be achieved between the client, family and professional members of the team, and those who may be briefly or tangentially involved.

- Documentation in the clinical record is essential.

2. ISSUES

Examination of client issues refers to assessed areas of impairment or concern which may require direct intervention, or may affect the outcome of proposed interventions.

For example:

- Progressive physical deterioration and irreversible swallowing dysfunction.

- Grieving for lost function and acceptance or denial of the terminal state.

- Understanding of the implication of reduced ability in eating and the options available.

- Cost and availability of feeding equipment.

3. MANAGEMENT OPTIONS

The team should establish priorities in treatment and collectively plan goals in management.[7] The client and family will often determine the course of treatment. There are three eating and feeding options available to the client:

3.1 NO INTERVENTION

The client elects to continue eating and drinking orally. Progressive deterioration in the ability to swallow will eventually result in weight loss and dehydration.

- Assistive devices, such as modified cutlery and head supports are offered.

- Staff and caregivers are encouraged to accept and support the client's wishes.

- Comfort measures, including suctioning and pain relief medication, are implemented.

3.2 MODIFICATIONS

Increasing difficulties with swallowing and feeding can be alleviated to a varying degree with planned modifications. Some which may be helpful are set out in heading form:

Swallowing [4,10]

- Swallowing routine.

- Assessed various head positions to minimise likelihood of aspiration.

- Supraglottic swallow.

- Suctioning routine.

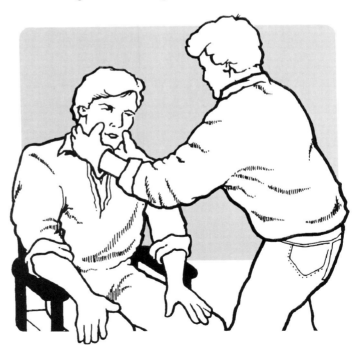

Eating

- Specific oro-facial muscle exercises.[7][10]

- Brushing and icing technique. [11]

- Denture re-line and oral hygiene routine.

- Modification to texture of food and fluids (see chapter 4)
e.g.: thickened fluids, non-chew semi-solid diet.

- Introduction of oral supplements either as partial snacks or complete meal replacements.

- Emphasise taste, temperature, smell and appearance of food offered.

Feeding

- Small and frequent meals.

- Supervised and private dining area.

- Food and fluid intake daily diary.

- Modified cutlery, such as lightweight enlarged grips and swivel cutlery.

- Modified crockery, such as 'Manoy' deep rimmed plates and plate-guards. [18]

- Stabilising crockery by use of 'Dycem' matting.

- Modified cup, mug or glass, e.g. lightweight beakers, 'Pat Saunders' straw.

- Modified positioning, e.g. winged headrest, splints and weights.[18]

- Visual feedback and cleaning routine, e.g. mirror or video.

- Preparation of appropriate foods, e.g. cook-freeze and proprietary foods.

3.3 ALTERNATIVE FEEDING

If the transition to alternative feeding is gradual, then palatable, nutritionally complete formulae can be given orally before tube feeding begins. Crisis introduction of alternative feeding occurs when the client is malnourished and dehydrated, and asks for active nutritional intervention.

Where the client's oral intake has diminished over a period of time, the gradual introduction of iso-osmolar, low fat formulae will be easiest to tolerate and quickest to empty from the stomach. The use of fibre - containing formulae will depend on the client's usual fibre intake and presence of constipation/diarrhoea. Small frequent volumes of formulae, foods or fluids should be offered when stomach capacity is reduced.

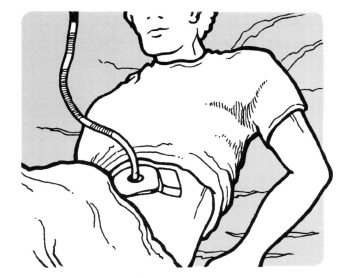

Options for alternative tube feeding differ according to the site of insertion, and have various pros and cons that require careful consideration. (See Chapter 4.)

Naso-Gastric [2,10,16,19]

+ Relatively easily inserted: does not require anaesthetic.

+ Immediate benefit to client.

+ Readily reversible.

- Visual and tactile irritation can lead to removal by client.

- Not appropriate where an obstruction exists between the nasal passages and upper esophagus.

- Possibility of gastric reflux and aspiration of stomach contents.

- Aesthetically distasteful to the client and visitors.

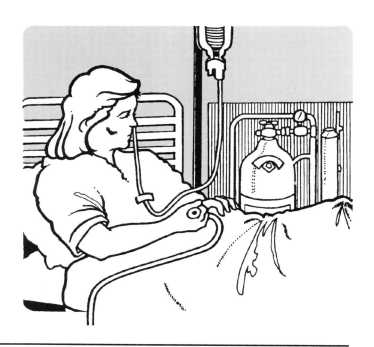

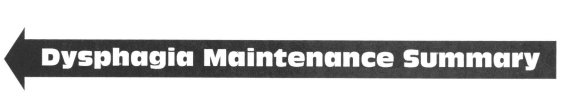

Dysphagia Maintenance Summary

Gastrostomy/Jejunostomy [2,5,12,19]

+ Cosmetically more appealing, as stoma site is easily concealed by clothing for aesthetic reasons.

+ More comfortable.

+ Reduces sensory irritation during administration of formula.

+ Increases normalisation and opportunities to socialise with family and friends.

+ Less likely to be accidentally removed.

+ Reversible procedure.

- Percutaneous endoscopic gastrostomy and jejunostomy procedures require at least a local anaesthetic and a minor surgical procedure.

- Risk of infection at stoma site and other complications (e.g. peritonitis).

- Other less likely operative risks include respiratory arrest and further medical complications if attempted late in the disease process.

Commonly, clients may receive daily nutrition and hydration requirements via alternative tube feeding and still enjoy with safety the taste and oral sensation of small amounts of suitable favourite food and fluids.

COMMON DISEASE CHARACTERISTICS

1. ADVANCED MOTOR NEURONE DISEASE (MND)— AMYOTROPHIC LATERAL SCLEROSIS (ALS)

1.1 ETIOLOGY [10,16,20,21]

Most cases of MND occur sporadically and with unknown cause. Viruses, metals, endogenous toxins, immune dysfunction, endocrine abnormalities, impaired DNA repair, altered axonal transport, and trauma have all been etiologically linked with MND, but convincing evidence of a causative role for any of these factors is yet to be demonstrated. A small percentage of cases are thought to be hereditary.

1.2 SYMPTOMS

Swallowing and eating [22,5,16]

• Poor lip closure is common.

• Difficulty with tongue control and oral manipulation of food and fluid develops. Bunching of the tongue through spasticity is common.

- Weakened chewing ability becomes progressively more prominent.

- Impaired velopharyngeal closure results in nasal regurgitation.

- Delayed swallow reflex and altered sensory feedback occur as the disease progresses.

- Saliva may be increased and more viscous, or lacking.

- Mouth infections, such as thrush, develop due to reduced oral phase activity.

- There is reduced laryngeal elevation and pharyngeal peristalsis.

- Cricopharyngeal muscle dysfunction occurs.

- Esophageal reflux is common.

- Reduced head control can create great difficulty in maintaining a comfortable and safe posture during meals.

Associated Characteristics [2,5,10,21]

- Initially asymmetrical weakness is evidenced by hand weakness or foot drop. In the later stages of the disease gross physical involvement of the upper and lower motor neurones renders clients functionally quadriplegic.

- Respiratory muscles become involved, resulting in inco-ordination and reduced vital capacity.

- Gradual loss of muscle mass due to reduced use may be unavoidable.

- Intellect and memory remain unaffected.

- Sensory involvement is rare.

- Eventual loss of expressive communication through speaking and writing poses great problems.

Prognosis [21,22,23]

The duration is dependent on the variant of MND, with bulbar presentation having a survival time of approximately 2 years. The average duration of the disease is 3-4 years, but there is wide variation in survival. Some cases seem to stay at a clinical plateau for months or even years, even though electromyographic and other studies may show covert continuing progression.

1.3 MANAGEMENT

Before alternative feeding

- Counselling, education and support from self-help groups, e.g. referral to Motor Neurone Society.

- Maintain function where possible, by using aids and devices to promote independence in eating and trying to reduce further complications, e.g. with a palatal lift prosthesis. [16]

- Establish a safe swallowing regime, e.g. specific exercises and routine to promote safe swallowing of food and fluids, namely muscle exercises and icing. [2,16]

- Symptomatic relief may be obtained via:

  * Increasing fluids, to reduce viscosity of the saliva.

  * Medication, such as Amitriptyline to reduce saliva. [22]

  * Surgery, such as ligation of the salivary ducts or cricopharyngeal myotomy, to improve specific aspects of swallowing. [10,16] However, in practice these procedures are rarely indicated or effective due to the deteriorating function of the whole swallowing mechanism.

- Support alternative therapy options e.g. natural herbs and remedies such as lemon juice and papaya enzyme, which are purported to reduce the viscosity of saliva.

- Introduce modifications to food texture and fluid consistency, e.g. thickened fluids and a vitamised main meal.

- Discuss and monitor changing food intake patterns and requirements with the client and family. Encourage them to be involved in planning the amount, frequency, timing and types of food and/or supplements that are offered.

- Promote good physical positioning to reduce the likelihood of aspiration or regurgitation of stomach contents. Determine suctioning requirements.

Indications for the introduction of alternative feeding as the main source of nutrition and hydration

Severely compromised nutritional status, e.g. significant malnutrition, with accompanying thirst and mental changes.

Severe dehydration.

Frequent aspiration and/or choking episodes made worse by copious, thick secretions.

- Reduced cough reflex and respiratory function, producing infections, including acute or recurrent aspiration pneumonia.

- Increasing fatigue and emotional exhaustion from repeated attempts at eating and drinking.

- The client requests a specific form of alternative feeding because of restricted oral intake.

- Administration of medications can be continued unobtrusively by this form of delivery.

Contraindications to the introduction of alternative feeding

- The client makes an informed decision not to elect for alternative nutrition and hydration.

- Medical condition progresses rapidly to a preterminal stage.

2. TRANSITIONAL FEEDING MANAGEMENT IN ADVANCED HUNTINGTON'S DISEASE (HUNTINGTON'S CHOREA)

2.1 ETIOLOGY [9,20,24]

Huntington's Disease (HD), also called Huntington's Chorea, is an inherited degenerative disorder that affects the basal ganglia and cerebral cortex. It is an autosomal dominant disease.

2.2 SYMPTOMS

Swallowing and eating [2,9,10]

- Unpredictable and sudden gulps of air during swallowing may cause aspiration and/or choking.

- The tongue becomes writhing (trumpet-like), making chewing and eating difficult.

- Co-ordination of swallowing becomes increasingly more difficult as choreiform movements increase.

- Food and liquids often travel through the mouth to the throat at unpredictable speeds.

- Coughing, drooling, regurgitation and vomiting occur more frequently as the disease progresses.

Associated Characteristics [9,21,25]

- Chorea is characterised by irregular, rapid, and involuntary movements of the limbs and axial muscles.

- The client is in constant motion.

- Intellectual problems (e.g. memory and problem-solving) usually progress into a profound dementia.

- Eventually there is loss of effective expressive communication despite characteristic irregular, quick, and jerky facial grimaces.

- At the advanced stage the client is bed/chair bound with little functional voluntary physical movement, and may be unable effectively to communicate verbally or non-verbally.

Prognosis [9,21]

The disease is usually fatal within 15 to 20 years of the initial presentation of symptoms in the second, third and fourth decades. There is a risk of suicide, as children of an affected parent have a 50 percent chance of inheriting the disease.

2.3 MANAGEMENT

Before alternative feeding

- Promote independence in feeding by providing the client with finger foods that do not require utensils, such as sandwiches, fruits and selected baby-teething foods. Weighted cuffs often steady limb movements, but may cause fatigue. [25]

- Messy eating and anti-social table manners may require the provision of protective clothing. Families will often ask for separate meal times to lessen embarrassment.

- Position for eating requires priority to reduce the likelihood of aspiration and/or choking. [2]

- Introduce alterations to texture such as minced or vitamised foods to compensate for reduced ability to chew.

- Thin fluids may be thickened with either 'Carobel' or 'Supercol U' thickening agents, but are often surprisingly well managed in the advanced stages of the disease.

- A typical swallowing routine will incorporate:

  * Placement of food in the mouth where the client takes the food off the spoon unaided.

  * Use of a plastic-coated spoon will help to prevent dental damage.

  * Reminder to the client to clear all food from the mouth before swallowing to prevent aspiration before the swallow.

- Head and limb restraint should be introduced with caution, as this will not reduce involuntary movements.[25] Feeders may best use the gentle force of their own arms and hands to steady head movements.

- Dietary considerations are important, as clients require a high energy intake to counterbalance energy used through constant movement.[10,13]

Intervention might include:

* Increasing frequency and volume of high energy meals;

* Provision of high energy oral supplements;

* Maintaining a daily food diary and fluid balance chart, for analysis, then identifying deficits and translating into appropriate amounts of food and drink items.

* Education on purchase and preparation of suitable snack foods;

* Maintaining a weekly weight chart.

- Support and counselling for the client and caregivers, and referral to Huntington's Disease Society, are often appreciated.

Indications for the introduction of alternative feeding as the main source of nutrition and hydration

- Severely compromised nutritional status, e.g. the client is emaciated and unable to satisfy hunger and nutrient needs by oral intake alone.

- Frequent episodes of choking and aspiration are exacerbated by reflux and vomiting of stomach contents on sudden, violent choreiform movements.

- Ability to feed with dignity and without forcible restraint is no longer possible.

- A legally competent client, or a person legally empowered to act on behalf of a legally incompetent client, asks for a specific form of alternative feeding because of restricted oral intake. This is rare in Huntington's Disease.

Contraindications to the introduction of alternative feeding

- A legally competent client, or a person legally empowered to act on behalf of a legally incompetent client, has made an informed decision not to accept alternative nutrition and hydration. In South Australia this matter may be covered by signing a declaration under the Natural Death Act. [31]

- Death is imminent and alternative feeding will not significantly improve quality of life, or may further complicate final existence.

3. TRANSITIONAL FEEDING IN ADVANCED PARKINSON'S DISEASE

3.1 ETIOLOGY

Parkinson's disease is associated with an idiopathic degeneration of the substantia nigra of the basal ganglia, resulting in a relative excess of cholinergic activity. [7, 21] The degree of dopamine deficiency correlates with the severity of the symptoms. [20] These may fluctuate considerably, producing the "on-off" phenomenon. A specific underlying cause has not been defined. [21]

3.2 SYMPTOMS

Swallowing and eating

- Tongue tremor may severely reduce the initiation of lingual movement in the oral phase. [14]

- There is often a markedly slowed oral transit time because of the repetitive anterior to posterior rolling pattern of the tongue ("tongue pumping"). The posterior tongue remains elevated, preventing food from leaving the oral cavity and resulting in drooling. [14, 26]

- A moderate delay in the swallow reflex is common.

- Reduced pharyngeal peristalsis with pooling in the valleculae and pyriform sinuses increases the risk of aspiration after the swallow. [14, 27]

- Incomplete laryngeal closure due to weakness in muscles elevating and pulling the larynx anteriorly during a swallow compromises airway protection.

- Cricopharyngeal spasm may result in vomiting and aspiration from spillover. [7, 14]

- Reduced esophageal peristalsis may be shown by cinefluography. [14]

Associated characteristics [7, 20, 26, 28]

- Rigidity is characterised by steady resistance to passive movement. Sometimes the rigidity is rhythmically jerky and is called 'cogwheeling'.

- Bradykinesia is delay or the inability to initiate, and reduction in the amplitude of voluntary movements, such as smiling.

- Resting tremor appears when the client is totally relaxed, and in the fingers or hands is described as 'pill-rolling'.

- Problems occur related to posture and adjustment of balance.

- Progressive loss of expressive communication occurs, e.g. writing, facial expression, intelligibility of speech.

- Dementia develops in approximately 15 to 20 percent of cases.

- Reactive depression is very common.

Prognosis

The onset of Parkinson's disease is usually in the sixth decade and over,[14] and progression varies greatly as the client acquires other conditions often seen in old people, e.g. degenerative joint disease.

Symptomatic management may include drug combinations of L-dopa and other agents to alleviate side-effects.[10, 26]

Because of the "on-off" phenomenon, the timing of medication and relationship to meals may be very important.

3.3 MANAGEMENT

Before Alternative Feeding

- Monitor timing of dopaminergic medications to ensure that their effect can facilitate oral and pharyngeal movements around meal-times.[10]

- Introduce aids and devices to promote independence in feeding, such as modified cutlery and crockery to compensate for movement disorder.

- Modifications to the daily meal plan may help compensate for excessive time taken to masticate food, e.g. small, frequent and highly nutritious meals.

- The texture of food requires little modification until the end stages of the disease, when introduction of a soft, minced or vitamised diet with supplements may help alleviate symptoms of fatigue and poor motivation. (see Chapter 4)

- Posture for eating requires monitoring to ensure adequate airway protection, especially when the client is being fed in the final stages of the disease.

- A typical swallowing routine may incorporate:

    * Increased sensory input of food and fluids (e.g. colour, increased smell and flavour) before mastication;

    * Placement of food on the posterior tongue with firm downward placement to trigger the swallow reflex. [2,10]

    * Double swallow followed by cough or throat-clearing to prevent aspiration of food particles after the swallow.

- Education, support and counselling of the client and caregivers can be assisted by a referral to the Parkinson's Syndrome Society.

Indications for the introduction of alternative feeding as the main source of nutrition and hydration.

- Daily nutrition and hydration requirements are unable to be met orally. Malnourishment and dehydration are the result of laboured and excessive time taken to eat.

- The final quality of life is complicated by frequent episodes of aspiration and/or choking, making eating no longer safe or dignified.

- Necessary medications can no longer be administered by mouth with reliability or good effect.

- A legally competent client or a person legally empowered to act on behalf of a legally incompetent client asks for active nutritional support.

Contraindications to the introduction of alternative feeding.

- A legally competent client or a person legally empowered to act on behalf of a legally incompetent client has made an informed decision not to accept alternative nutrition and hydration. In South Australia this matter may be covered by signing a declaration under the Natural Death Act. [31]

- The client is able to maintain adequate daily nutrition and hydration needs through eating, albeit slowed.

- The client is in a pre-terminal state with death impending.

4. TRANSITIONAL FEEDING MANAGEMENT IN ADVANCED MULTIPLE SCLEROSIS (M.S.)

4.1 ETIOLOGY [7,21]

This disease is characterised by variable-sized plaques of demyelinisation, which can occur anywhere in the white matter of the central nervous system, but classically peripheral nerves are not affected. A specific cause has not been confirmed.

4.2 SYMPTOMS

Swallowing and eating

Because lesions in the brainstem may affect pathways to single or multiple cranial nerves, the resultant interference with swallowing can be of varying types. [9, 10]

- Glossopharyngeal (IX) cranial nerve involvement will result in a delayed swallow reflex and possibly reduction in pharyngeal peristalsis.

- Vagal (X) cranial nerve involvement will compromise laryngeal function to some extent (e.g. reduced vocal cord adduction). Airway protection and the risk of aspiration are then a concern.

- Hypoglossal (XII) cranial nerve involvement will result in weakness of tongue muscles and functional mastication.

Associated characteristics

The nature of the neurologic deficits in M.S. will depend on the location and the size of the demyelinating plaques. No two clients are the same. [2,29,30]

- Muscular weakness and spasticity of the lower extremities are often accompanied by painful flexor spasms, requiring continuing medication. [21]

- Gait and limb ataxia reduce independence, and the latter can seriously interfere with independent feeding.

- As the disease advances there will be varying degrees of spastic paralysis, producing hemiparesis, paraparesis, quadriparesis, and (rarely) monoparesis. [21, 30]

- In the late stages there is usually eventual decline in expressive communication through one or more of: [2,10]

  * Ataxic spastic dysarthria;

  * Reduced neuromuscular co-ordination for respiration;

  * Impaired vital capacity;

  * Organic dementia or other profound defects from extensive demyelination.

- Visual disturbance can occur from involvement of the optic nerve, the central pathways, and internuclear ophthalmoplegia affecting convergence and accommodation. [21, 30]

- Cognitive impairment may be shown by memory loss and difficulties with new learning and conceptualisation. [30]

- Depression, denial and euphoria may also be manifestations of the disease, and of the emotional response to it. [21]

Prognosis [9,21,30]

Symptoms usually begin in early or middle adult life, and the course varies from a few years to apparent arrest with fixed disability and otherwise normal ageing. Evolution of disability is clearly related to the progressive phases of the disease, for the course is often staccato, with temporary or permanent, partial or complete return of function depending on the location and activity of the demyelinating process.

4.3 MANAGEMENT

Before alternative feeding

- Positional changes (head flexion) will help to prevent aspiration before the swallow.

- Promote independence in eating with modified utensils, crockery and upper extremity orthotics, such as a weighted forearm cuff to reduce the effects of ataxia, or splinting.

- Ensure removal of distractions to eating and encourage adequate speed of eating. [2]

- Specific oral muscle strengthening exercises may help maintain tongue motion, strength and control. [10]

- A typical swallowing routine may incorporate:

  * Increased cognitive awareness of eating through sensory input, such as smell, colour and texture.

  * Teaching the client to overchew and develop a purposeful supra-glottic swallow (i.e. inhale and hold breath at the height of inspiration and then swallow).

  * Coughing on exhalation after the swallow to expectorate residue in the pharynx or upper airway.

- Introduce modifications to food texture and fluid consistency to reduce oral fatigue e.g. by a non-chew diet with thickened fluids and high energy formulae such as 'Ensure Plus' and 'Sustain'.

- Monitor nutritional status and nutrient requirements, especially during periods of exacerbation or febrile illness.

- Encourage small, varied and frequent meals.

- Offer counselling, education and support, including referral to the Multiple Sclerosis Society. [29, 30]

Indications for the introduction of alternative feeding as the main source of nutrition and hydration

- Acute exacerbation of the symptoms temporarily prevents adequate oral intake of food and fluids. [10]

- Chronic malnutrition and dehydration have developed, being common at the end stage of the disease.

- A legally competent client, or a person legally empowered to act on behalf of a legally incompetent client, asks for a specific form of alternative feeding because of restricted intake. This is rare in advanced multiple sclerosis.

Contraindications to the introduction of alternative feeding

- A legally competent client, or a person legally empowered to act on behalf of a legally incompetent client, has made an informed decision not to accept alternative nutrition and hydration. In South Australia this matter may be covered by signing a declaration under the Natural Death Act. [31]

- The client has an acute exacerbation which is starting to resolve.

- The client has entered a pre-terminal stage and death is imminent.

CHAPTER 2 REFERENCES
Transition from eating to alternative feeding

1. Donner M. *Swallowing mechanism and neuromuscular disorder.* Semin Roentgenol 1974; 9: 273-82.
2. Groher ME (ed). *Dysphagia: diagnosis and management.* Boston: Butterworths, 1984.
3. McIntosh J, Martin G, Sacchett C. *Recognition of the diverse and complex nature of neuromuscular swallowing disorders: a basis for treatment.* Clin Rehabil 1987 ; 1: 39-45.
4. Miller RM, Groher ME. *The evaluation and management of neuromuscular and mechanical swallowing disorders.* Dysarth Dysphon Dysphag 1982 ; 1: 50-70.
5. Goldblatt D. *Treatment of amyotrophic lateral sclerosis.* Adv. Neurol 1977 ; 17: 265-83.
6. Warfel JH, Schlagenhauff RE. *Understanding neurologic disease: a textbook for therapists.* Baltimore: Urban and Schwarzenberg, 1980
7. Romine JS. *Demyelinating disorders.* In: Wiederhold W.C. Neurology for non-neurologists New York: Academic Press, 1982.
8. Walsh TM. *Disease of nerve and muscle.* In: Samuals M A. *Manual of Neurologic Therapeutics.* Boston : Little, Brown & Co ,1982.
9. Cherney LR, Cantieri CA, Pannell JJ. *Clinical evaluation of dysphagia.* Maryland: An Aspen Publication, 1986.
10. Logemann J. *Evaluation and treatment of swallowing disorders.* San Diego: College-Hill Press Inc ,1983.
11. Morrell RM. *Neurolgic disorders of swallowing.* In: Groher M.E. (ed). *Dysphagia: diagnosis and management.* Boston: Butterworths, 1984.
12. Steefel J. *Dysphagia rehabilitation for neurologically impaired adults.* Springfield: Charles C. Thomas, 1981.
13. Daly D, Code C, Anderson M. *Disturbances of swallowing and esophageal motility in patients with multiple sclerosis.* Neurology 1962 ; 12: 250-6.
14. Donner M, Silbiger M. *Cinefluorographic analysis of pharyngeal swallowing in neuromuscular disorders.* Am. J. Med. Sc. 1966; 251: 600-16.
15. Welnetz K. *Maintaining adequate nutrition and hydration in the dysphagic A.L.S. patient.* Can Nurs 1983; 3: 30-4.
16. Cochrane GM (ed). *The management of motor neurone disease.* U.K.: Longman Group U.K. Ltd., 1987.
17. Scheinberg L, Smith CR. *Rehabilitation of patients with multiple sclerosis.* Neurol Clin 1987 ; 5: 585-600.
18. Farber SD. *Neurorehabilitation: a multisensory approach.* Philadelphia: W B. Saunders,1982.
19. Annas GJ. *Do feeding tubes have more rights than patients?* Hastings Centre Report 1986 Feb: 26-8.
20. Lechtenberg R. *The psychiatrist's guide to disease of the nervous system.* New York: Wiley,1982.
21. Prater RJ, Swift RW. *Manual of voice therapy.* Boston : Little, Brown & Co ,1984.
22. Newrick PG, Langton-Hewer R. *Motor neurone disease: can we do better? A study of 42 patients.* Br Med J 1984; 289: 539-42.
23. Rose FC (ed). *Motor neurone disease.* London : Pitman Medical Publishing Ltd ,1977.
24. Klawans HL, Goetz CG, Perlik S. *Presymptomatic and early detection in Huntington's disease.* Ann Neurol 1980: 8: 343.
25. Leopold NA, Kagel MC. *Dysphagia in Huntington's disease.* Arch Neurol 1985; 42:157-60.
26. Lieberman AM, Horowitz L, Redmond P, Pachter L, Lieberman I, Leibowitz M. *Dysphagia in Parkinson's Disease.* Am J Gastroenterol 1980; 74 :157-60.

27. Palmer ED. *Dysphagia in Parkinsonism.* JAMA 1974; 229 :1349.

28. Logemann J, Blonsky E, Boshes B. *Dysphagia in Parkinsonism.* JAMA 1975; 231: 69-70.

29. Delisa JA, Miller MM Milkulic M, Hammond MC. *Multiple sclerosis:part II common functional problems in rehabilitation.* Am Fam Physician 1985; 32 :127-32.

30. Hallpike JF. *Multiple sclerosis: modern management.* Patient Manag 1987; Jul :155-64.

31. Natural Death Act 1983, *No. 121 of 1983.* D.B. Dunstan, Governor, South Australia.

3

TRANSITION FROM ALTERNATIVE FEEDING TO EATING

Partial or complete neurological dysphagia commonly occurs after cerebral trauma, such as head injury and cerebral infarction.[1,2,3] When referred for assessment and swallow rehabilitation clients are usually already receiving alternative nutrition.

The aims of intervention are to determine the client's readiness to commence eating with safety and to achieve maximum independence with confidence. A comprehensive team assessment will define the client's strengths and deficits. The management plan will incorporate achievable short term goals to facilitate improvement in swallowing or to compensate for lost function. The long term goal is not to offer what may be an unrealistic guarantee of outcome, but instead to provide an estimation of potential functional ability.

It must be clearly understood and accepted by all concerned, especially family members, that a transitional feeding program in this setting can be time-consuming, frustrating for all involved, and slow-moving. Rehabilitation of a swallow following severe or complex brain trauma is often measured in weeks and sometimes months.

TEAM MEMBER ROLES

Rehabilitation of swallowing dysfunction requires the skills of a multidisciplinary team drawn from medicine, nursing, the allied health professions, and dentistry. Family members are viewed as equal participants. The composition of the team will alter according to the client's rate of recovery and priority needs in the overall rehabilitation program.

The extent of involvement of different professions and the tempo of activity differ from the situation in progressive disease. The roles and relationships described below have been very successfully developed at Julia Farr Centre, but there will naturally be variations elsewhere.

FAMILY

Family members are usually very anxious to be involved from the earliest opportunity, and should be encouraged to do so. Problems can arise from difficulty in accepting (to the point of complete rejection or denial) the risks of premature oral feeding. Much time and patience are required in maintaining support and good relationships in this setting, especially as conflicts over eating can have multiplier counter-therapeutic effects in other parts of the rehabilitation program.

SPEECH PATHOLOGIST

Undertakes specialist assessment, diagnosis and management of swallowing dysfunction. In many institutions the speech pathologist is the team leader in swallow rehabilitation. This role encompasses education, evaluation and co-ordination of the multidisciplinary team.

DIETITIAN

Monitors the client's overall nutritional status and intake, making recommendations on daily requirements. As an essential resource person the dietitian liaises between catering staff and the speech pathologist to ensure appropriate provision of nutritious foods and fluids of a prescribed texture and consistency.

MEDICAL OFFICER

Establishes (if necessary with specialist help) the anatomical and physiological basis for the difficulty with swallowing, monitors progress (especially potential complications, such as aspiration and dehydration), ensures continuity of medication during the transitional feeding program, and provides professional authority to reinforce the actions and advice of other staff.

NURSE

Has closest contact with the family, provides nursing care, monitors the client's overall state and vital signs, implements prescribed eating and alternative feeding programs, and attends to respiratory and oral hygiene.

PHYSIOTHERAPIST

Conducts an assessment of overall physical and respiratory function, including advice on tracheostomy care, suctioning requirements, posture, and safety techniques.

OCCUPATIONAL THERAPIST

Assesses manual feeding skills, provides adaptive equipment, assesses perceptual and cognitive factors, and provides technical skills and advises on positioning at meal times.

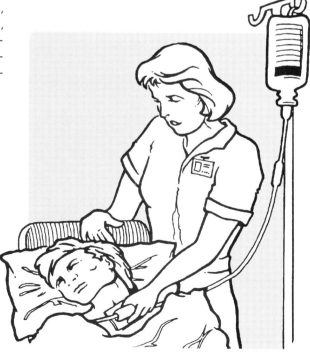

SOCIAL WORKER

Supports and counsels the client and family and may adopt a mediating or advocacy role should there be conflict.

DENTIST

Provides overall assessment of dental status including oral hygiene, denture fit, gum disease and developing caries; participates in management of local trauma (such as fractured

mandible), provides preventive dentistry; may provide velo-pharyngeal pros-
theses; and at the request of treating staff may provide a mouth guard to
reduce likelihood of oral trauma due to hypertonic bite reflex.

CLINICAL PSYCHOLOGIST

Participates in cognitive assessment and directs a behavioural management
program in appropriate clients with aggressive or other behavioural difficulties.

Note:

> Roles of individual team members may differ between institutions, home-
> care facilities, different states and countries. Often roles will merge
> depending on the emphasis of the service and individual skills and expe-
> rience of team members.

ASSESSMENT AND EVALUATION

Early referral and assessment after cerebral trauma are most useful in establishing a first approximation of the time that may be taken to achieve recovery, or
at least a plateau state. Usually the client can give little information, and that
provided by the family may not be complete or accurate.

If the client has been transferred from an acute hospital for rehabilitation elsewhere it is essential that all clinical narrative records be available to the professional team responsible for taking over management. Summaries and discharge letters are inadequate and may not be accurate or up-to-date.

There are four main areas to be evaluated:

1. Medical condition, especially neurological status.
2. Status before eating.
3. Eating and swallowing.
4. Independence - eating and feeding.

1. MEDICAL CONDITION

Evaluation of the client's neurological condition is conducted as part of a general medical examination and aims to determine where the lesions are, what
the lesions are, their functional consequences, and the degree to which other
neurological and psychological factors may affect rehabilitation potential.

Other medical issues, such as fractures and abdominal surgery must be clearly
defined.

*The examination involves assessment of the most important factors relevant to
a transitional feeding program:*

1.1 THE HIGHER FUNCTIONS [4,5,6,7]

Cerebrum, namely level of consciousness, behaviour, emotional state,
thought processes and specific localised cerebral functions, such as paralysis,

apraxia, aphasia, agnosia and paresis.

Cranial Nerves, in particular the trigeminal (V),facial (VII), glossopharyngeal (IX), vagus (X), and hypoglossal (XII).

Cerebellum, such as ataxia and intention tremor.

1.2 THE MOTOR SYSTEM

Evaluation involves comparisons of tone, power, range of movement, wasting and tremor or fasciculation, with particular reference to the upper limbs.

1.3 THE SENSORY SYSTEM

Perception of touch, pain, temperature, taste and vibration are evaluated.

2. STATUS BEFORE EATING

The process of initial assessment can be time consuming and require a number of sessions over several weeks. (See Assessment Flowchart, page 13)

2.1 COGNITIVE LEVEL

Routine neurological observations, such as the Glasgow Coma Scale give a clear indication of lightening in conscious state and the tempo of recovery. The Glasgow Coma Scale and Rancho Los Amigos Scale should be very strongly encouraged, to allow comparison between progress and outcome of each client, and of groups of clients in the same and different institutions. (See Factors Affecting Outcome, page 128)

It is essential that a thorough multidisciplinary assessment is undertaken to confirm stability of conscious state to avoid premature and potentially dangerous introduction of oral intake.

Other factors to be investigated include:

- Attention span.

- Concentration—vigilance—effort.

- Awareness—insight—motivation.

2.2 RESPIRATORY STATUS

If there is a recent history of respiratory complications, it is essential to clarify and to document for all involved in management:

- Tracheostomy requirements: i.e. type (e.g. cuffed, un-cuffed), model (e.g. pediatric, fenestrated) and effectiveness in situ. Pulmonary and oro-pharyngeal suctioning requirements. [8]

- Air entry, usual findings on auscultation, and expansion.

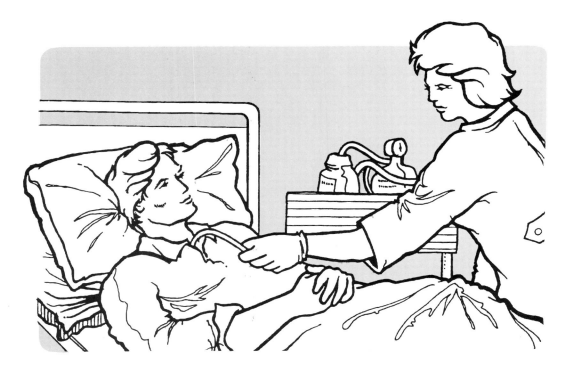

- Effectiveness of the protective cough reflex and subsequent sputum management. Risk of aspiration and/or choking on oral secretions. (See Aspiration, Choking and Emergency Procedure, Chapter 5.)

2.3 PROTECTIVE REFLEXES [3,6,10]

Before commencing eating and drinking, a client should possess certain functional reflexes that will protect the airway and ensure maximum safety during swallowing:

- Gag Reflex - response stimulates strong contraction of the pharyngeal wall and soft palate resulting in forward propulsion to clear the pharynx.

- Swallow Reflex - response initiates the non-volitional velo-pharyngeal/pharyngeal stage of swallow.

- Cough Reflex - response helps clear the airway of irritating substances and mucous, as the diaphragm contracts, larynx elevates and pharynx constricts. Note that the voluntary cough and cough reflex are neurologically independent of one another. [3]

Assessment is undertaken of swallowing, both spontaneous and volitional (i.e. in response to command) to determine the effectiveness of the swallow and attempted compensation for impaired function.

It should be noted that of these three reflexes only the swallowing reflex and cough reflex are essential for safe oral intake. The presence or absence of a gag reflex cannot determine swallowing proficiency as each of these reflexes is neurologically independent (i.e. presence or absence of one does not necessarily indicate the presence or absence of any of the others). [3]

2.4 ORAL REFLEXES

As a result of bilateral frontal lobe damage, oral reflexes of two types may be observed and interfere with normal swallowing patterns: [2,9]

- Abnormal reflexes at any age that directly interfere with attempts to eat, such as bite and tongue thrust reflexes.

- Primitive reflexes usually associated with infantile eating patterns may actually assist in swallow rehabilitation. This apparently paradoxical principle applies to suck-swallow, mouth-opening and rooting reflexes.

2.5 PHYSICAL STATUS

This should incorporate examination of:

- Head control.

- Upper limb function, i.e. co-ordination, active motor function, range of movement, tone and contractures.

- Sitting balance.

2.6 PERCEPTUAL AND SENSORY ABILITY

- Visual field deficit.

- Visual neglect.

- Distance, depth and colour perception.

- Sensitivity to taste, smell, touch, vibration, temperature, kinaesthesia and pain.

2.7 COMMUNICATION

This requires assessment of:

- Functional ability to follow verbal and written instructions.

- Functional expression via speech or writing to enable feedback during the rehabilitation process.

3. EATING AND SWALLOWING

The dysphagia assessment is conducted by a speech pathologist. Extreme care must be taken to ensure the safety of the client throughout the eating portion of the assessment, which requires food and fluid to be placed in the mouth.

3.1 EVALUATION OF PERIPHERAL SPEECH MECHANISMS AND ORAL MOTOR FUNCTION

The clinician begins with an examination of muscle function, noting slowness, completeness of performance, and overall co-ordination, by assessing: [6,10,11]

- Facial musculature at rest, e.g. asymmetry and drooling.

- Lips, e.g. asymmetry and poor closure.

- Teeth, e.g. loose fitting dentures and poor dental hygiene.

- Tongue, e.g. deviation, reduced rate and range of movement.

- Jaw, e.g. inability to align teeth.

- Palate, e.g. deviation and reduced velopharyngeal closure.

- Laryngeal musculature, e.g. reduced upward movement of larynx.

- Glottal closure, e.g. weak reflexive or volitional cough.

- Taste, e.g. inability to differentiate salt, sour, sweet or bitter tastes.

3.2 EVALUATION OF SWALLOWING ABILITY THROUGH INTRODUCTION OF TRIAL EATING TECHNIQUES

This phase of assessment is graded in complexity and potential difficulty for the client. For this reason, it is essential for the client to demonstrate success (with minimal distress) at each level before progressing to the next. Failure to progress to the next level indicates that the client is 'at risk' for example from a compromised protective cough reflex, abnormal oral reflexes, or a severely reduced swallow reflex.

Further evaluation of swallowing beyond the level assessed to be safe requires consultation with the medical officer to discuss the issue of liability, potential for aspiration and resultant complications.

Level 1: Evaluation of Dry Swallow

The clinician should:

- Examine reflexive swallow of the client's own saliva, noting the number of swallows over a 10 minute period (the normal figure is between 5 and 10).

- Elicit a volitional swallow on command by asking the client to swallow, noting what cueing or prompts are required to do so.

- Compare any differences or delay between volitional and voluntary swallows.

CHECKLIST for ALTERNATIVE FEEDING to EATING

IMPROVING FUNCTION

 ADEQUATE PROTECTION OF AIRWAY

- Productive cough reflex

or
- Cuffed tracheostomy tube

or
- Compensatory head and neck position to reduce likelihood of aspiration or choking.

 REASONABLE STABILITY IN CONSCIOUS STATE

- The client can stay awake for at least 20 - 30 minutes.
- The client demonstrates consistent awareness of the environment and responds to procedures.
- Cognitive scales:
  Santa Clara Valley - Advanced Primary Level
  Rancho Los Amigos - Level 2/3 - 4 (8)
  Glasgow Coma Scale - Level 9 (15)

 STABILITY IN MEDICAL AND NUTRITIONAL STATUS

- The major current clinical emphasis is on rehabilitation rather than dealing with an acute situation or complication.

 ORAL PHASE IS ADEQUATE FOR SWALLOWING

- Degree of functional lip and tongue movement is adequate for mastication and/or bolus transport from lips to pharynx

and
- Abnormal oral reflexes (eg: bite, tongue thrust) have reduced and facial sensitivity is normalising

and
- Stimulable swallow reflex
  ARE ALL PRESENT.

 ESTABLISHED MANAGEMENT SUPPORT SYSTEM

- Caregivers (family and otherwise) are educated and support the transitional feeding program.
- The client is motivated to improve swallowing and overall function.
- All caregivers (including family) are confident with emergency aspiration and choking procedures, which are clearly documented.

Note: Impairment in communication does not preclude beginning a transitional feeding program.

A lemon swab squeezed dry and placed in the mouth can assist in the initiation of a swallow at both levels, should saliva be sparse.

Level 2: Evaluation of swallowing function with trial oral intake of food and fluid with specified textures.

Under no circumstances should this level of assessment be undertaken until the client has been confirmed to be stable in conscious state and to have cough and swallow reflexes.

Safety is paramount. All involved (including family members) must feel confident with positioning, what to do for choking, and how to undertake suction. There must be no distractions for the client or for the caregivers (professional and family).

When the client is adequately prepared the evaluation should begin with:

1. **Semi-solid texture**, for example low acid jelly or baby gel.

Rationale

* This texture is easily expectorated if it enters the airway, which it should not occlude. [12]

* It stimulates the `anticipatory phase' of a swallow.

* It allows for the `preparatory phase' of eating, through placement and extra time to initiate chewing movements.

* It is unlikely to be aspirated before the swallow without rotary chewing movements to propel the bolus backward, in contrast to fluids, which may easily escape posteriorly without mastication.

Instructions

* Have the client take ½ teaspoon of gel from the spoon, using lip closure around the spoon if possible. Otherwise place the gel on the middle portion of the tongue with a firm downward movement.

* Ask the client to chew the bolus and swallow in the normal way.

Evaluation

* The clinician should carefully note the effectiveness of the swallow reflex, any evidence of aspiration or client distress, and regurgitation or spillage from the mouth.

SUMMARY

WNL *(Within Normal Limits)*		*Degree of* *Difficulty*		*No Function* *Discontinue Assessment*
X	X	X	X	X
	LOW	MED	HIGH	

2. **Fluid consistency**, for example free and thickened fluids.

Rationale

* Clients on prolonged tube feeds will often complain of thirst and dryness in the mouth. [13]

* In practice free fluids are much more difficult to manage and swallow than semi-solids, and are the single most likely cause of aspiration if given before expert assessment of competency.

Instructions

* The clinician should offer the client either ½ teaspoon of water or icechips, and encourage lip closure and a supraglottic swallow (i.e. hold breath, followed by swallow).

* If difficulty is noted with free fluids, they may be thickened and assessed in the same way.

Evaluation

* Observation should reveal any evidence of aspiration, drooling or nasal regurgitation.

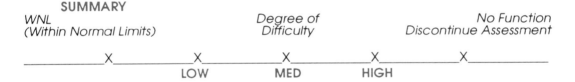

SUMMARY

WNL (Within Normal Limits)	Degree of Difficulty	No Function Discontinue Assessment

X   X   X   X   X

LOW   MED   HIGH

3. **Chew texture**, such as minced, soft and solid food options.

Rationale

* When the client has been assessed to be competent with semi-solids the potential ability with more difficult food types may be assessed.

* In swallow rehabilitation clients will often begin eating a vitamised diet for safety and fatigue reasons. The natural progression to foods requiring increased chewing ability will be faster for some clients than others, depending on individual needs and capabilities.

Instructions

* The client is offered ½ teaspoon of food requiring increased chew, such as mashed vegetables and mashed banana. The client is asked to "overchew" and to undertake a supraglottic swallow.

* If a minced texture succeeds, soft and then hard foods may be evaluated in the same way.

Evaluation

* The clinician should note the quality of chewing, oral transit time (i.e. time taken to chew and initiate a swallow) any evidence of aspiration before, during and after the swallow, nasal regurgitation or spillage from the mouth.

SUMMARY

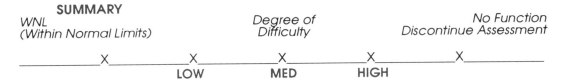

WNL — *Degree of* — *No Function*
(Within Normal Limits) — *Difficulty* — *Discontinue Assessment*

LOW   MED   HIGH

Evaluation and re-evaluation can be a time consuming and often repetitive task.

Other factors to take into account during assessment include:

● Procedures after assessment, such as to ensure that the client sits upright for at least thirty minutes after a trial of oral intake.

● The possibility of silent aspiration without clinical symptoms or signs. [2,3] The respiratory state and temperature chart must be closely followed.

● Use of radiological examination. A chest x-ray may reveal evidence of aspiration, and contrast cinefluography is strongly recommended if there is doubt of laryngeal/pharyngeal/esophageal phase dysfunction.

Cine or video-fluoroscopy of swallowing is a technique which involves recording the passage of radio opaque material such as barium in a liquid, semi-solid or solid form through the pharynx, esophagus and stomach.[3] This form of assessment is best done in consultation with the speech pathologist, radiologist, and dysphagia team. Although quick and relatively safe these results are only meaningful when detailed clinical examinations of Before Eating and Eating status have been conducted beforehand.
Cinefluoroscopy may not only confirm the presence of dysphagia and/or aspiration, but also assist in future therapeutic strategies and recommendations.

4. INDEPENDENCE IN EATING AND FEEDING

Assessment of independence in eating and feeding involves direct evaluation of:

4.1 POSITIONING

This requires considering: [14]

● Head, arm and hand posture and functional movements in relation to placement of food and drink.

● Functional upper limb movements for self feeding (assisted and unassisted).

- Furniture in the dining area, e.g. wheelchair at table, tray on wheelchair, or overbed table in bed.

The effects of visual inattention, visual field deficit or body neglect.

4.2 PREPARATION AND FEEDING

This requires considering: [14,15]

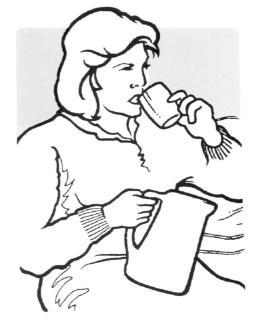

- Food preferences and eating habits to enable appropriate ordering of food.

- Choice of suitable cutlery and crockery.

- The client's awareness, concentration and distractibility.

- The use of protective garments, such as a feeding apron.

- The need for splinting or other supports, such as cushions or a head rest.

- Level of supervision and prompting.

- Oral hygiene regime. [27]

- Acceptable feeding time limits with planned alternatives such as replacement tube feed.

- Monitoring levels of motivation, fatigue, frustration, fear of eating.

INTERVENTION

The aim of swallow rehabilitation is the safe and efficient oral intake of food and fluids with maximum independence and quality of eating and drinking. A gradual transition from alternative feeding to eating orally as the main source of nutrition and hydration (without undue nutritional, medical or emotional distress) is the goal of this phase of management.

A clear, objective description of the client's presenting strengths and delineation of issues in management is required for the team to set priorities, and to give an estimate of the duration of treatment.

Members of the team should agree on realistic goals, both in the short term and more remotely. Once again we stress the necessity to closely involve the family in doing so.

1. STRENGTHS

This means assessed areas of ability that can be built upon in management.

For example:

- The client is motivated and able to follow simple instructions.

- The client has good oral hygiene and dentition.

- The client recognises errors and attempts to self-correct.

- The client has a functional upper limb which may be used for self-feeding.

2. ISSUES

This refers to assessed areas of dysfunction or concern, which require intervention or which may affect outcome.

For example:

- Abnormal oral reflexes preclude normal eating patterns.

- The client has poor or inconsistent awareness and attention, resulting in distractibility.

- The client is grieving for lost function and is depressed and unmotivated or actively resisting therapies.

3. MANAGEMENT OPTIONS

Preliminary planning should incorporate:

- Contingency planning to develop alternative strategies when desired change or progress is not achieved.

- Reinforcement techniques, including verbal prompting, cueing and progress charts.

- Feedback and documentation.

- Appropriate staffing levels, education, and motivation for implementation of the transitional feeding program.

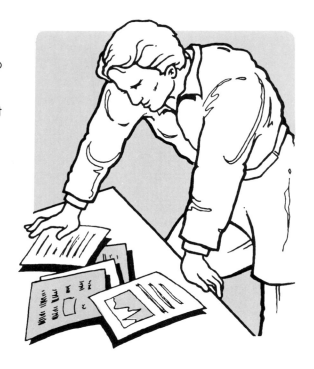

- Regular review meetings to discuss the results of interventions.

The factors involved in assessing a client's readiness to undertake swallow rehabilitation are summarised in the 'Alternative feeding to eating checklist' mentioned earlier in this chapter. (page 57)

The results of assessment will determine the level of intervention:

3.1 NO INTERVENTION

The client is not ready to begin a transitional feeding program.

- Continue alternative nutrition.

- Nil intake by mouth, including medications.

- Recommend re-evaluation after an agreed interval.

3.2 INTERVENTION BEFORE EATING BEGINS

If the client has corrigible deficits these are attended to as a matter of priority. It should be agreed by the team that no eating trials will be undertaken until this has been done.

Cognitive status.

Environmental sensory stimulation and specific techniques are used to enhance attention to time, task and person.

Respiratory status.[16]

The cough reflex is stimulated to try to clear the chest. Expert advice may be sought to confirm whether a different type of tracheostomy tube is required. (See Aspiration, Choking and Emergency Procedures, Chapter 5.)

Abnormal oral reflexes.

As the conscious state improves, the desensitisation techniques described in chapter 6 may help to reduce abnormal oral reflexes if they are interfering with successful eating.

Physical status.

Preliminary intervention may involve head and neck strengthening exercises, and postural changes from lying to sitting upright while supported. Postural adjustment should inhibit abnormal tone and whole body reflex patterns such as asymmetrical tonic neck reflex (ATNR).

Perceptual and sensory ability.

Intervention may include stimulation of touch, smell and hearing. If there is a hemianopia the client may be helped to compensate for the loss by learning to track across the midline and to achieve compensatory scanning.

Communication ability.

Where possible a reliable form of Yes/No communication or valid feedback system (verbal or non-verbal) is of great advantage.

Oral muscle status.

Specific exercises may be prescribed for the client to improve oral muscle functioning before eating. Compensation for weakness or inco-ordination may be achieved through daily oro-motor muscle exercises involving the rate, range and strength of lip, tongue, palate, face and jaw muscles. (See chapter 6.) Such neuromuscular treatment exercises involving inhibitory and desensitizing stimulation for hypersensitivity, hypertonicity and hyperreflexia, and excitatory stimulation and strengthening for hyposensitivity, hypotonicity, and hyporeflexia must be prescribed by a speech pathologist or physiotherapist. Such exercises are generally followed by a functional eating and/or movement task and if used without the latter have little or no benefit to the client.

3.3 EATING INTERVENTION

When the client has been assessed to be ready for oral intake, the speech pathologist initiates a period of rehearsal. This is an instructional phase during which the client is helped to use those techniques which trials have shown to help achieve an effective swallow.

Rehearsal Level

- Demonstrate safety procedures to the client, such as suctioning and the cough-swallow technique.

- Demonstrate and have the client practice a safe swallowing routine without, and then with, food placed in the mouth, namely:

  * Check posture and positioning.

  * Ensure that there is an appropriate amount and texture of bolus and that it is correctly placed on the tongue.

  * Encourage the client to close the lips around the spoon.

  * Instruct the client to pause and bring the head forward (chin on chest) to protect the airway.

  * The clinician should model and have the client imitate a strong 'plunge swallow'.

  * Ask the client to cough or phonate 'ah' after the swallow, to evaluate evidence of aspiration, namely a gurgly voice or audible noises in the laryngeal area.

- Practice facilitatory swallow techniques, such as specific swallow reflex stimulation through temperature, taste and texture; the overchew technique; supraglottic swallow, or two stage swallow.

- Determine the ability to learn and maintain newly taught skills in swallowing. This will be directly affected by fatigue and motivational factors, and will in turn determine the degree of supervision, cueing and prompting required.

- Evaluate episodes of aspiration, how aware the client is of errors, and how much the client attempts to self-correct.

- Continue to increase tolerance, the goal being to swallow about 6 teaspoonsful in a session lasting ten minutes. It may take several sessions to achieve this.

Eating Levels

When the client becomes adept at swallowing semi-solids at the rehearsal level, the transition to eating may commence.

1. To begin with, the client is supervised by the speech pathologist and usually requires considerable prompting and reinforcement.

   - The goal of eating rehabilitation at this level is to achieve ⅓ - ½ cup (80-120mls) of trial texture three times per day with little or no difficulty. Food and fluid balance charts are helpful to chart progress. Evaluation of feeding versus independent eating should also be conducted at this level.

   - No alterations should be made to the tube feeding regime at this stage.

2. When the client achieves a consistent and reliable trial intake of semi-solids three times daily, trained team members (including family) may become involved in feeding and supervision of swallowing.

   - The goal of eating rehabilitation at this level is to introduce small portion meals of the trial texture, e.g. vitamised main meal and dessert. Initially the client may only manage one small meal per day and will gradually build-up tolerance to two and three meals a day. Previous eating preferences, habits and fluctuations in eating performance at this level must be considered in planning meals. It is wise to document the times in which maximum oral intake is achieved in order to determine eating trends and 'best meal time'.

     Any difficulties in eating and swallowing must all be carefully documented as well.

- Once the client is able to manage eating at this level, the speech pathologist should introduce a safe fluid intake. However if the initial assessments indicate little or no difficulty with fluid intake, fluids of a specified thickness may be introduced even before trials with semi-solids.

Where possible it is best that the client learns to drink from a cup in the normal way. The progression is made from teaspoon to either straw or cup.

Note:

For some clients spouted beakers should be avoided as they encourage head extension during swallowing.

- Alteration in the tube feeding regime is required to accommodate an increasing oral intake of foods. Aim to encourage hunger and appetite without compromising nutritional status.

  * Intermittent feeding and catch up feeds at night may be considered to establish an eating pattern based on normal meal times.

  * Spacing of supplementary tube feeds around oral meal times to encourage hunger.

  * Offer preferred foods initially, acceptance of complete meals may be delayed.

  * Reduce volume of tube feeding formulae to achieve an energy deficit to stimulate hunger. The amount of energy deficit is dependent on the anticipated tempo or duration of transitional feeding.

Eating rehabilitation nears completion when the client manages the best potential texture (e.g. minced, soft, solid) of food and fluids with little or no difficulty. A maintenance level of supervision and prompting is then agreed. Ensure that regular reviews and re-evaluations are planned to ensure that the client's safest texture is upgraded as spontaneous improvement occurs.

The client is now able to maintain daily nutrient and fluid requirements by mouth. Particular attention to consistent fluid intake is necessary as this may fluctuate with variations in motivation, fatigue and increasing physical and cognitive requirements. Formulae may be given orally to supplement energy intake if required. Providing nutritional assessment shows adequate intake of variety and appropriate quantities of the different food groups as well as energy and fluids, food and fluid charts may no longer be required. Adequate intake is required to achieve and maintain ideal weight.

Tube feeding should now be withdrawn.

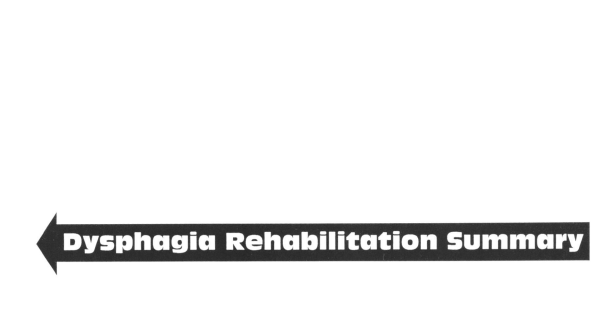

Dysphagia Rehabilitation Summary

Some clients will never achieve safe independence in eating and may:

- Always require maximum supervision and prompting.

- Plateau at a certain level (e.g. thickened fluids) and not progress any further.

- Require help with feeding indefinitely, as their physical ability does not allow for safe independence in eating.

- Present with persistent eating and swallowing difficulties despite concentrated rehabilitation attempts. Consideration should then be given to surgical or prosthetic management (i.e. a swallowing device), and the ethics of recreational eating with specific textures or favourite snack foods.

3.4 FEEDING INTERVENTION

Maximum independence in both eating and feeding may be achieved through: [3,14,17]

- Provision of modified cutlery e.g. a 'rocker' knife to cut food one handed with a rocking rather than sawing action.

- Provision of modified crockery, e.g. a perspex plate guard to assist with forking up the food. Stabilising crockery, e.g. 'Dycem' matting or clamps.

- Provision of a modified drinking vessel, e.g. a lightweight see-through cup to allow the client to watch drinking.

- Modified positioning, e.g. a winged head rest, or splints.

- A visual feedback and cleaning routine, e.g. to use a mirror, and wash cloth.

This graded and comprehensive approach to swallow rehabilitation has an emphasis on safety, efficiency and maximum independence in eating and feeding. It helps to determine the level of maximum improvement and when to terminate treatment.

SEVERE TRAUMA

1. TRANSITIONAL FEEDING AFTER TRAUMATIC BRAIN INJURY

1.1 CLINICAL FEATURES

Manifestations vary according to the location and extent of the brain injury and the presence of associated pathology, such as fractures of the facial bones and upper limbs.

Swallowing and Eating

- If both frontal lobes are affected the client will revert to primitive and/or abnormal oral reflexes. [2, 4]

- Spasticity or weakness of the tongue produces difficulty with tongue control and the oral manipulation of food. [3, 4]

- If the swallow reflex is delayed there is a risk of aspiration before, during, and after the swallow.

- Drooling may result from poor lip closure.

- Palatal movement is often limited.

- Mouth infections such as thrush develop, due to a reduced oral phase.

- Cricopharyngeal dysfunction may occur. [2, 3, 4,]

- Esophageal reflux must be considered. [18]

Associated Characteristics

- Significant motor impairment: [14, 19, 20]

  * Severe spasticity is usual after major brain injury.

  * Loss of motor control occurs in any or all four limbs.

  * There is impaired head and trunk control.

  * The client is completely dependent in activities of daily living.

- Significant impairment in perceptual skills:

  * Poor visual attention and scanning limit the client's ability to co-operate. [20]

  * Dyspraxic motor planning deficits arise when there is damage to the parietal connections.

  * Clients often have poor fine and gross visual and perceptual motor skills.

  * Cerebellar deficits are very common. [20] Those involving the vermis and its connections produce truncal ataxia, with difficulty maintaining sitting balance for feeding. Involvement of lateral connections produces intention tremor, which can be intensely frustrating and produce embarrassment from messy eating. [9]

- Significant cognitive and behavioural impairment:

  * Post Traumatic Amnesia and memory deficit are universal in severe brain injury.[7]

  * The client usually has poor awareness and insight, cannot solve simple problems, perseverates, and readily fatigues.[14]

  * The client develops manipulative behaviours, such as screaming and active resistance.

- Significant respiratory impairment: [8,11,21]

  * The client often still has a tracheostomy, management of which can interrupt attempts at feeding and distract the client and caregiver (especially a family member, see page 116)

- Severe communication impairment: [6,22]

  * Severe brain injury usually produces a varying combination of expressive and receptive dysphasia, dysarthria and dyspraxia.

1.2 MANAGEMENT

Before Eating

- Much time and effort, and sometimes great patience, are required to give counselling, education and support to the client and caregivers, both nurses and family.

- Respiratory precautions are essential and the methylene blue test is a helpful guide in clients with tracheostomy (see page 117).[2,3]

- Compensate for severe language impairment by simulating familiar eating routines, food preferences, and personal habits.

- Encourage an upright symmetrical posture progressing from assisted to unassisted head control.

- The environment should be free from distractions so that all involved can concentrate on the program.

- Introduce short periods of concentration and attention to tasks, such as orientation to time, place and person, visual tracking and focussing.

- If there are problems with aggressive behaviour, techniques such as differential reinforcement and situational "time-out" may help to achieve better behaviour at mealtimes.

Eating

- Specific oro-facial muscle exercises are valuable.

- Brushing and icing techniques help to reduce spasticity.

- Desensitisation procedures are applied for abnormal oral reflexes.

- The swallow reflex is stimulated by such means as temperature (hot/cold) and varying tastes (e.g. chilli, fondant) and texture (e.g. 'Whizz Fizz', lollipops).[23]

- Maximum sensory stimulation is presented during eating by sight and smell.

- Promote normalisation in eating very early in the rehabilitation program, from lip closure around the spoon and normal drinking from a cup to maximum independence in self-feeding. [14]

- Use simple verbal cues and instructions to avoid confusion or hesitation.

- Establish a safe swallowing routine with an array of successful facilitators, such as model swallow, assisted laryngeal swallow through manipulation of the larynx, overchew and 'plunge' swallow.[2,3,6]

- Compensate for deficits in initiation and self-feeding by consistent and gentle physical and verbal prompting.

- Introduce adaptive equipment to promote maximum independence, such as crockery, non-skid pads, drinking cups, utensils and splinting.

- Introduce self-monitoring through visual feedback and cleaning routine.

- Monitor fatigue and ensure frequent, brief training sessions.

- Encourage a routine of good oral hygiene. [27]

2. TRANSITIONAL FEEDING AFTER SEVERE CEREBROVASCULAR ACCIDENT (C.V.A.)

2.1 PHYSICAL SIGNS

These will vary according to the location and extent of interruption to cortical activity:

LEFT HEMISPHERE (DOMINANT) LESION

Swallowing and Eating [2,3,6,24]

- The client will usually show contralateral reductions in lip and tongue strength, rate and range of movement, and sensation.

- A delayed swallow reflex is common.

- Contralateral reductions in pharyngeal peristalsis may occur.

Associated Characteristics [10,14,25]

- Expressive and receptive language impairment are very common.

- Motor speech and motor planning disorders may arise.

- There is a right hemiplegia or hemiparesis.

- Reactive depression is understandable and often overlooked or underestimated.

RIGHT HEMISPHERE (NON-DOMINANT) LESION

Swallowing and Eating [2,10,11,13]

- There may be contralateral reductions in lip and tongue strength, rate and range of movement and sensation.

- A delayed swallow reflex may occur.

- There may be contralateral reductions in pharyngeal peristalsis.

Associated Characteristics [10,13,14]

- The neuromuscular symptoms are compounded as it is more difficult to use compensatory techniques because of reduced orientation, deficits in perception and attention, errors in judgement with impulsivity, and loss of intellectual control over swallowing. The most extreme form of this phenomenon is denial of disability (anisognosia).

- The client usually has a left hemiplegia or hemiparesis.

BILATERAL HEMISPHERE LESIONS

Swallowing and Eating [2,12,13]

- The client shows reduced tongue and lip strength, rate and range of movement, and sensation.

- The swallow reflex is delayed.

- Reduced pharyngeal peristalsis occurs.

- Chronic aspiration is a continuing hazard.

- Cricopharyngeal involvement may occur.

Associated Characteristics [25,26]

- The client will usually revert to abnormal or primitive oral reflexes.

- There is spasticity and loss of motor control in any or all four limbs.

- Cognitive, perceptual, communication and behavioural manifestations may preclude good functional compensation for a swallowing deficit.

BRAINSTEM LESION

Swallowing and Eating [2,12,13,21]

- Lip and tongue movements are reduced in rate, range and strength, and there may be associated sensory impairment.

- The swallow reflex is absent or delayed.

- Pharyngeal peristalsis is reduced.

- Reduced laryngeal adduction may occur.

- Cricopharyngeal spasm may be present.

Associated Characteristics [2,18]

- Severe respiratory crisis can develop, necessitating interim or chronic tracheostomy or ventilatory support.

- Aspiration of sputum requires a suctioning regime.

- Severe depression is an understandable response, especially when cognition is relatively intact (the "locked in" syndrome).

- Minimal, if any, motor, perceptual, cognitive or communication deficit.

2.2 MANAGEMENT

Before Eating

- Counsel, educate and support the client and family.

- Compensate for language impairment by simulating familiar eating routines, food preferences, and personal habits.

- Compensate for contralateral limb paralysis and weakness through correct posture and positioning.

- Ensure that there is an optimal environment for re-learning swallowing and eating patterns.

- Encourage early independence in self-feeding by utilising function in an unaffected upper limb.

- Introduce short, frequent training sessions according to fatigue, pre-morbid ability and motivation.

Eating

- Ensure good oral hygiene [27] and denture fit.

- Employ specific oro-facial muscle exercises and brushing and icing techniques.

- Stimulate the swallow reflex by variations in temperature, taste and texture.

- Try to exploit sight and smell to achieve maximum sensory stimulation during eating.

- Encourage early independence with dignity by providing assistive devices.

- Monitor perceived motivation and chart progress to help to reinforce the client's determination to improve.

- Establish a safe swallowing routine and determine the level of supervision required for eating and drinking.

- Monitor awareness of errors and attempts to self-correct incorrect eating patterns.

- Introduce favourite foods and drinks as goals in progress.

CHAPTER 3 REFERENCES
Transition from alternative feeding to eating

1. Donner M, *Swallowing mechanism and neuromuscular disorder.* Semin Roentgenol 1974;9:273-82
2. Groher ME (ed), *Dysphagia: diagnosis and management.* Boston: Butterworths, 1984.
3. Logemann J. *Evaluation and treatment of swallowing disorders.* San Diego: College-Hill Press Inc.,1983.
4. Cherney LR, Cantieri CA, Pannell JJ. *Clinical evaluation of dysphagia.* Maryland: An Aspen Publication, 1986.
5. Chusid JG. *Correlative neuroanatomy and functional neurology.* 16th ed Los Altos: Lange,1976.
6. Steefel J, *Dysphagia rehabilitation for neurologically impaired adults.* Springfield: Charles C. Thomas, 1981.
7. Warfel JH, Schlagenhauff RE. *Understanding neurologic disease: a textbook for therapists.* Baltimore: Urban and Schwarzenberg, 1980.
8. Cameron JL, Reynolds J, Zuidema GD. *Aspiration in patients with tracheostomies.* Surg Gynecol Obstet 1973 ; 136: 68-70.
9. Lazarus C, Logemann JA. *Swallowing disorders in closed head trauma patients.* Arch Phys Med Rehabil 1987; 68: 79-84.
10. Miller RM Groher ME. *The evaluation and management of neuromuscular and mechanical swallowing disorders.* Dysarth Dysphon Dysphag 1982; 1: 50-70.
11. Morrell RM. *Neurologic disorders of swallowing* In: Groher M.E. (ed) Dysphagia: diagnosis and management. Boston: Butterworths, 1984
12. Veis SL, Logemann JA. *The nature of swallowing disorders in CVA patients.* Arch Phys Med Rehabil 1985; 66: 372-5.
13. Gordon C, Hewer RL, Wade DT, *Dysphagia in acute stroke.* Br Med J 1987; 295: 411-14.
14. Farber SD.*Neurorehabilitation: a multisensory approach.* Philadelphia:W.B Saunders, 1982.
15. McIntosh J, Martin G, Sacchett C. *Recognition of the diverse and complex nature of neuromuscular swallowing disorders: a basis for treatment.* Clin Rehabil 1987 ; 1: 39-45.
16. Selley WG. *Swallowing difficulties in stroke patients: a new treatment.* Age Aging 1984 ; 14 : 361-5.
17. Olivares L, Segovia A, Revuelta R. *Tube feeding and lethal aspiration in neurological patients: a review of 720 autopsy cases.* Stroke 1974; 5: 654-7.
18. Clifton GL Robertson CS, Choi SC. *Assessment of nutritional requirements of head injured patients.* J. Neurosurg 1986; 64: 895-901.
19. Dinning TAR, Connelly JJ. *Head injuries—an integrated approach.* Brisbane: John Wiley & Sons, 1981.
20. Kalisky, Z Morrison DF, Meyers CA. *Medical problems encountered during rehabilitation of patients with head injury.* Arch Phys Med Rehabil 1985; 66: 25-9.
21. Ehberg D, Nylander G. *Cineradiography of the pharyngeal stage of deglutition in 250 patients with dysphagia.* Br J Radiol 1982; 55: 258-62.
22. Prater RJ, Swift RW. *Manual of voice therapy.* Boston : Little, Brown & Co ,1984.
23. Mansson 1, Sandberg N, *Salivary stimulus and swallowing reflex in man.* Acta Otolaryngol 1975;79:445-50.
24. Meadows J, *Dysphagia in unilateral cerebral lesions* J Neurol Neurosurg Psychiatry 1973;36:853-60.

25. Axelsson K, Norberg A, Asplund K. *Relearning to eat late after a stroke by systematic nursing intervention: a case report.* J. Adv Nurs 1986; 11: 553-9.

26. Broe GA. *Parkinsonism and related disorders.* In: Caird Fl. (ed) *Neurologic disorders in the elderly.* Bristol: Wright, 1982.

27. Gryst MEI, *An oral hygiene manual for the caregivers of disabled people,* Adelaide: Julia Farr Centre Foundation, 1990

NUTRITION
AND
ALTERNATIVE
FEEDING

Nutrition is the science of food in relation to both the physical and the emotional needs of the human body.

Client centred nutrition involves the individual assessment of daily food and fluid intake, comparing it with requirements, planning suitable intervention, facilitating the implementation of strategies and evaluating its success.[1] With the dysphagic person this may involve food modification for easy swallowing and provision of acceptable nutritious drinks. Where possible the client needs to feel in control of his or her choices.

Optimum success can be achieved by following a process of: [1]

- Assessing requirements
- Planning intervention
- Implementing strategies
- Evaluating progress

1. ASSESSING REQUIREMENTS

Nutritional requirements are assessed by relevant team members according to the clients' physical and mental condition and medical treatment.

Medical Examination

This is performed by the medical officer of the team and one of the aims is to highlight medical conditions requiring dietary intervention.

Medical examination provides:

- A description of the presenting trauma or complaint including onset, site of trauma or neurological lesion, typical characteristics and anticipated progression.

- The presence or anticipation of complications and their current and probable treatment.

- A review of current and past sources of medication and a detailed account of the past medical history, such as surgery, trauma, drug use. Drug-nutrient interactions involving commonly used medication such as phenytoin, antibiotics, analgesics, antacids, mono-amine oxidase inhibitors, and laxatives, should be considered. 2,3,4

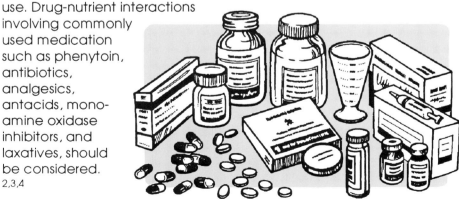

Note: Certain enteral formulae may interfere with or enhance drug absorption.

- A thorough topographical examination for symptoms and signs of malnutrition, with confirmatory investigations where necessary, including baseline studies for subsequent comparison in order to assess progress.

- An examination of physiological function of major organs, muscle action or rigidity and ventilatory capacity and identification of probable hormone imbalances.

Obtain Diet History:

A diet history is the unique tool of the dietitian and forms the basis for nutrition counselling. Information may be obtained from an initial interview on admission with the client on a 'typical' day. Variations to the pattern for weekends, when at home, or an admission to a nominated place for care, are taken into account. An alternative method of obtaining progressive information is to use a food diary or intake chart. The use of both historical and progressive methods provides the clinician with information on previous food intake patterns and eating behaviour, and allows comparison with current intake before and after counselling. When the client is unable to be interviewed, information on previous food intake patterns and eating behaviours can be obtained from family members. To elicit current general food behaviours, information obtained includes:

- Level of education

- Socio-economic status

- General health attitudes, beliefs and practices in relation to food

- Level of physical activity

- Nutrition knowledge

- Family support available

- Skill level of person responsible for food purchase and preparation

- Availability of time saving food preparation equipment

Information on specific food behaviours includes:

- Interview to recall 24 hour type and quantity of food intake.

- Attitudes to foods when eaten or avoided

- Food frequency check list

- Food likes and dislikes

- Taste preferences, i.e. sweet, savoury, spicy

- Appetite

Identify Nutrient Requirements

Recommended Dietary Intake

This provides a mean daily intake of each nutrient to ensure that minimum requirements to maintain a healthy body are being met. Conditions that elevate requirements are considered to avoid malnutrition.

Physiological Systems

- Assimilation of nutrients requires adequate digestion and absorption capacity. Factors affecting gastrointestinal digestion and/or absorption [5,6] will determine the efficiency with which proteins/fats/ carbohydrates are broken down and become useful to the body. Some commercial products provide nutrients in a predigested form which may assist this process.

- Elevated muscle activity associated with conditions such as hypertonicity, chronic uncontrolled movements or reduced ventilatory capacity (often in association with increased mucous production) will often elevate protein and energy requirements.

- Hormonal imbalances due to stress, trauma, surgery, burns catabolism, sepsis and abnormal body temperatures elevate energy requirements. [7,8,9]

- Electrolyte and fluid imbalances due to fluctuations in renal function, hormone production and drugs, especially diuretics must be considered. [10]

- Medical conditions requiring dietary intervention such as diabetes, renal failure, pancreatitis will alter the form (level of predigestion) and proportion of specific nutrients.

Protein requirements can be estimated either from recommended dietary intake (0.8gm per kg body weight, in Australia)[11] plus the additional effects of burns, trauma, injury, fever, stress and losses from sweat, urine and mucous. The other method is to determine nitrogen losses from urinary urea, convert this to protein and aim for a positive nitrogen balance from dietary sources.

Energy requirements can be estimated either from recommended energy allowance for body weight and age, then adjusted for activity,[12,13] or using formulae such as the Harris Benedict Equation for estimating basal energy expenditure plus the additional effects of extent of injury or trauma and activity level.

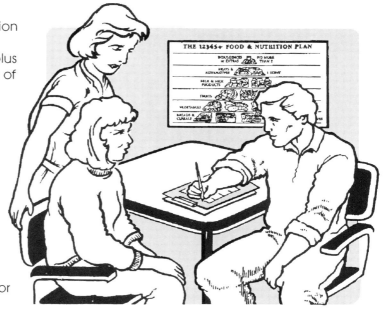

2. PLAN INTERVENTION

Once the nutritional needs of the client have been clearly identified the clinician and client establish specific goals. From these goals, objectives for changing behaviour or food intake are developed. The objectives are clearly explained to the client and family to facilitate understanding and motivation to learn. They may involve specific food texture modifications for safe swallowing and new eating patterns to meet requirements, as well as a change in balance of nutrients. [14]

2.1 DESIGN EDUCATION STRATEGIES

Education which involves change needs to be preceded by gentle investigation of barriers to change. [15] Examples of this are:

- Food aversions. These will be picked up in the diet history and counselling may be necessary.

- Grief. A level of acceptance needs to be reached before education on dietary changes can be effective.

Nutrition education tools are available for general information (food groups, dietary guidelines) or for specific dietary disorders (overweight, diabetic, renal failure). Often general nutrition information is suitable with modifications to meet some of the clients' objectives, while specific information may be available from specialist organisations or support groups. Designing one's own educational material, while rewarding, is often time consuming. The following are examples of educational tools found useful in the education of clients and family in transitional feeding.

Nutrient Adequacy:

Foods with similar nutrients are often grouped together into food groups. The amounts to be eaten from each group ensure that the recommended

12345+
Food and Nutrition Plan

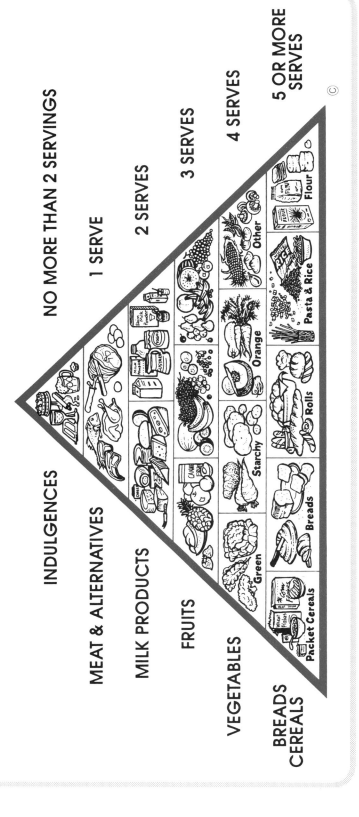

INDULGENCES — NO MORE THAN 2 SERVINGS

MEAT & ALTERNATIVES — 1 SERVE

MILK PRODUCTS — 2 SERVES

FRUITS — 3 SERVES

VEGETABLES — 4 SERVES
Green · Starchy · Orange · Other

BREADS CEREALS — 5 OR MORE SERVES
Packet Cereals · Breads · Rolls · Pasta & Rice · Flour

©

daily intake of specific nutrients can be met. For example, the "**12345+ food and nutrition plan**" developed by the CSIRO in Adelaide meets the recommended daily intake of all nutrients.[16]

This program addresses the issues of reducing the chronic disease profile of the community at large and encompasses current dietary recommendations of increasing breads and cereals, fruits and vegetables while lowering fat, sugar and salt. To meet different energy requirements it is suggested that the bread/cereal serve recommendations be adjusted (hence 5+). For growth and increased protein requirements an increase in meat and milk serves may be necessary.

Food Group	Recommended Amount		Nutrients Provided
Meat	1 serve	ie; 60-100gm lean red meat	Protein, fat, iron, magnesium, zinc, cholesterol, B12, thiamin, riboflavin.
Dairy	2 serves	ie; 40gm cheese, 200gm yoghurt 300 mls milk	Protein, Carbohydrates (lactose), calcium, zinc, cholesterol, riboflavin, sodium.
Fruit	3 serves	ie; medium piece fruit, 100 ml fruit juice	Fibre, natural sugars, folate, C, B6, magnesium, potassium, Beta-Carotene.
Vegetables	4 serves	ie; 1 potato, one-half cup green, one-third cup orange, one-third cup other vegetables	Fibre, folate A, C, iron.
Cereals (wholegrain)	5 + serves	ie; 1 slice bread (plus 1 tsp margarine), one-half cup cooked rice, 30gm packet cereal, 1 muffin, 1 cup cooked pasta	Protein, fibre, complex carbohydrates, fats, magnesium, zinc, iron, folate, B vitamins, sodium, Vitamin E (from margarine)

Sample Meal Plan -

	Modifications to Texture
Breakfast	
30gm wholegrain packet cereal Half cup milk Fruit or juice 1 slice wholemeal toast with jam/marmalade/honey	Soak softened cereal in warm milk. Puree fruit or thicken juice. Soak toast, blend with smooth spread and serve in ramekin.
1 slice wholemeal toast with cheese/mushroom/ tomato/baked beans/ scrambled egg Tea/Coffee	Add bread/toast crumbs to hot moist items and blend or mash at table with a fork. Thicken drink.
Morning Tea	
Biscuit/slice of cake	Plain cake set in jelly or served with custard.
Tea/Coffee	Thicken drink.
Lunch	
1 cup vegetabie soup Sandwich made with wholemeal bread	Thick pureed vegetables. Remove crusts. Use soft paste type fillings and cook in oven covered with beaten egg and milk.
Fruit	Puree fruit.
Afternoon Tea	
Fruit Scones/Muffins/Crumpet	Puree fruit. Soak cereal and process with smooth spread or fruit.
Tea/Coffee	Thicken drink.
Dinner	
2 slices roast meat/fish chicken	Blend or chop finely, top with soft pastry (mix ⅓ flour, ⅓ cottage cheese, ⅓ butter) serve with sauce or gravy.
1 potato ½ cup green vegetables ⅓ cup orange vegetables	Mash vegetables.
Fruit Icecream/Custard	Puree fruit. Not modified
Supper	
Milk drink	Thicken drink.

Adapted from Backhouse and Martin. [17]

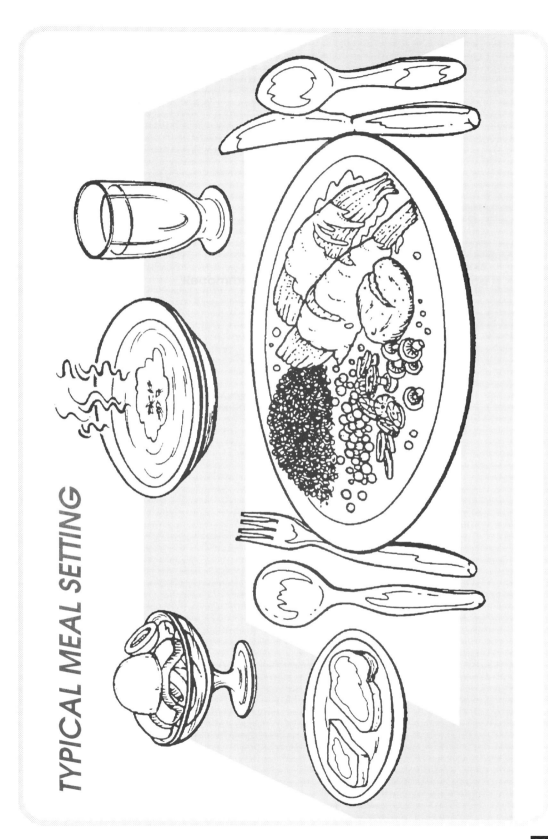

TYPICAL MEAL SETTING

85

Individual Meal Plans

A dietitian can design in conjunction with the client and family a 'typical' day's intake including main meals, snacks and drinks. This provides a reference for selecting recipes and illustrates what foods to select and how to balance their intake throughout the day. The clients in the institutional setting may be encouraged to select their own daily menu from a set plan. A food diary maintained at home by either the client or family on foods eaten, any difficulties experienced, and amount eaten, will assist the dietitian in reinforcing appropriate food choices and suggesting modifications.

Food Purchase and Preparation

The level of involvement by the team will depend on the clients' abilities and their previous experience or reliance on family members for food purchase and preparation. Specialist organisations and support groups can offer information booklets, recipe books and educational videos relevant to specific conditions. Purchasing appropriate pre-prepared or commercial food suitable with minimum preparation can save effort in the kitchen with little effect on nutritional content. The therapist may also investigate the use of time saving devices such as food processors and blenders. Acceptability of foods can be improved by adapting usual cooking methods to suit the clients' new needs.

Where the clients or family are unfamiliar with cooking, the use of illustrated step-by-step cook books is beneficial in gaining confidence. Practicing these new skills in a safe environment can be achieved with individual skills training by occupational therapists or skilled dietitians and home economists.

Modified Texture

The constituents of food have chemical and physical properties that give them different texture characteristics such as crunchiness, viscosity, consistency, adhesiveness, chewiness etc. Each of these properties vary on a continuum and for practical purposes we break textures into distinct groups or diets.

A speech pathologist can assess a person's swallowing ability and determine the food texture that is safest for the client. To assist the client and family in learning how to obtain foods of the desired texture the clinician may either use comprehensive lists of suitable foods, some of which will require processing, or describe methods of testing the appropriateness of foods with or without modifications for the required food texture.

An excellent resource is the recent publication "Good Looking, Easy Swallowing. (Creative Catering for Modified Texture Diets)." by Jane Backhouse and Janet Martin.[17]

The following are examples of food and fluid texture tests and suitable foods developed in conjunction with a speech pathologist:

VITAMISED/PUREED/SMOOTH & THICK

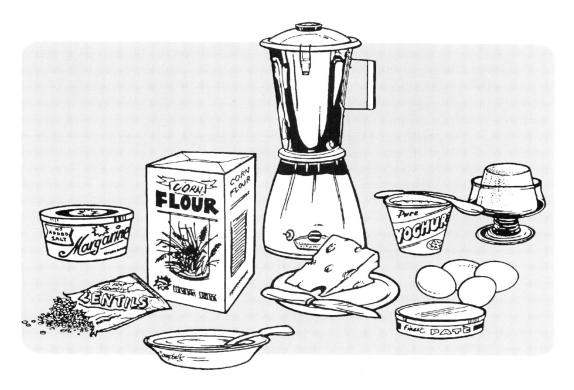

Test:

Smooth, with no hard lumps present, while thick enough to form furrows with the flat end of a spoon. Note that some may have a soft grainy/beady texture like cooked sago.

Examples include:

- Porridge pureed
- "Weetbix" soaked in milk
- Sago, tapioca cooked
- Flour, cornstarch to thicken sauces
- Pureed tinned/stewed fruit
- Soft vegetables pureed
- Melted cheese
- Icecream, custard, yoghurt (no lumps)
- Salmon mousse (in gelatin)
- Vitamised soft cooked meat in gravy
- Creamy scrambled eggs

MINCED/NON-CHEW/EASY CHEW

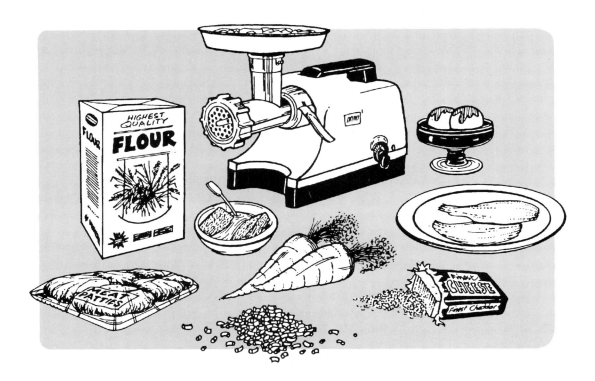

Test:

Can be broken up easily with the flat edge of a fork into 0.5cm pieces and should be thoroughly coated with a thick sauce.

Examples include:

- Porridge
- "Weetbix" soaked in milk
- Flour, cornstarch to thicken sauces
- Cut-up pasta,lasagna or spaghetti
- Rice mixed with thick sauce
- Finely cut tinned/stewed fruit
- Finely cut soft vegetables
- Melted soft crumbly cheeses
- Icecream,custard,yoghurt (no lumps)
- Poached or steamed fish
- Minced meats with thick gravy
- Finely cut meat & vegetables in stew or mornay

SOFT/BITE SIZED

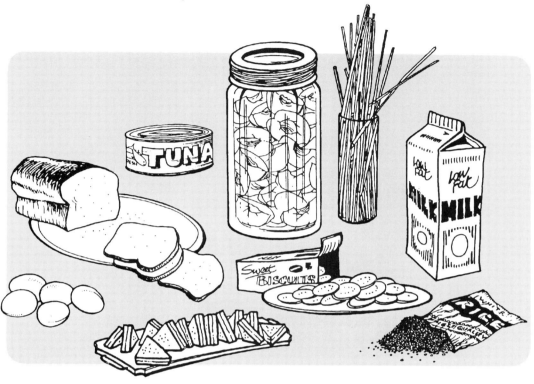

Test:
Can be broken into 1.5cm pieces with the flat edge of a fork.

Examples include:

- Soft breakfast cereals soaked in milk
- Sandwiches (no crust) with soft fillings e.g. egg, soft cheese, thin meat, tuna, salmon
- Soft biscuits.
- Pasta, rice
- Pastry
- Any well-cooked vegetable
- Fruits stewed or tinned
- All dairy products
- Stewed or casseroled meat pieces & vegetables
- Boiled or poached eggs

Ward Diet

A ward diet implies that the client can cope with all types of food and fluid consistencies without special modifications.

Thick Fluids

To test the consistency of thick fluids a line drawn into the surface should slowly disappear. Thin fluids may be thickened with starches (tapioca, sago, arrowroot, cornflour) or gums (agar agar, gelatin, guar gum). Instant commercial thickeners are also available in starches (`pregel-n`, `instant gel it`, `thick and easy`, `Liquiset`) and gums (`carobel`, `supercol-u`, `carboxy-methyl-cellulose`, `ketrol`) from the food industry.

2.2 PLAN NUTRIENT SOURCES

We obtain nutrients from a combination of foods and fluids that are consumed throughout the day. Adequate nutrition can generally be obtained from everyday foods and fluids provided the texture is safe and the client can eat the required amounts from each food group. Clients who are unable to meet their nutritional needs adequately from common foods or fluids may prefer to use nutrient dense drinks or complete supplements.

Foods

Foods are the preferable choice of providing nutrition as they are physiologically normal. They are also relatively cheap, readily available, vary in flavour, texture and offer limitless potential for combining to produce new flavours, aromas, and textures utilising naturally occurring starches and fibres.

Food challenges the imagination of both clinician, client and family and provides a means for improving the clients' quality of life. However, food choices may be limited due to client preferences, greater fatigue levels, difficulty preparing meals (time constraints, away from home), in which case supplements provide an easy alternative source of nutrition.

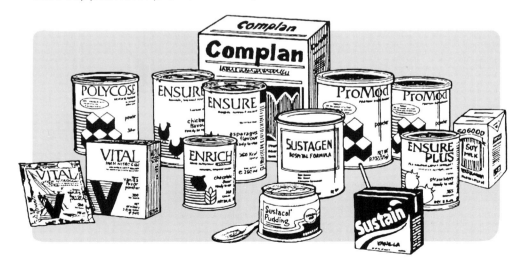

Supplements

Supplements are used to make it easier for clients to increase their intake of specific nutrients or as partial or complete meal replacements. Supplements vary in their palatability and it is often time-saving to provide a range of supplements for the client to taste. Supplements are available in the following forms:

- Vitamins and minerals as capsules or syrups.
  These can be difficult to swallow; this may be made easier by thickening syrups or encasing capsules in jelly or mixing with food.

- Protein powders, either as intact proteins such as whey/casein, or as amino acids (note excessive intake of protein can impair renal function and increase calcium excretion).[18]

- Fat, either as long chain fatty acids or medium chain triglycerides (MCT oil) which is readily absorbed. (Note excessive intake of fat is associated with obesity, and an increased risk of cancer and cardiovascular disease.)[19]

- Carbohydrates, either in the form of refined sugars, polysaccharides or polymeric sugars such as 'polycose'/'polyjoule', or unrefined as gums or starches for use as thickeners or dietary fibre.

- Semi/complete formulae are commercially produced to meet the nutritional needs of specific medical conditions or as meal replacements.

- Some supplements may be used in conjunction with or added to foods with little taste variation, thus providing a greater range of flavours and textures.

Intervention planning aims to develop a nutritional care plan which clearly outlines ways clients can meet their assessed nutritional needs as independently as possible. The following checklist is an example of developing a nutritional care plan:[1]

Client needs
- Ideal weight
- Improved food intake
- Food preparation skills/nutrition knowledge
- Assistance in food purchase/preparation

Client goals
- To achieve ideal weight
- To improve food preparation skills
- To increase variety of meals
- To arrange assistance in food purchase/preparation

Client objectives	• Reading educational material
	• Viewing relevant videos
	• Contact support groups
	• Provide recipes to trial with aim of trying 1 new recipe per week
	• Taste test of supplements
	• Practice using food processor
	• Incorporating breads and cereals into recipes
	• Use of daily meal plan for purchasing and preparing food
	• Contingency plan if meal not eaten
	• Maintain food diary

3. IMPLEMENT STRATEGIES

The successful implementation of a nutritional care plan requires a combined or team approach from relevant members of the health care team and family.

3.1 FACILITATE CLIENT LEARNING

An understanding of the clients' level of comprehension and preferred style of learning is important in achieving acceptance of new skills and knowledge. The teachers need to be flexible and adaptable in their teaching methods to meet the needs of the client. Learning involves motivation and acceptance of new ideas, and then an opportunity for the client to practice these new skills in a relaxed environment. Client learning can be enhanced by education of family members in order that they may reinforce new skills and knowledge and provide support in the home environment.

Information presentation may be facilitated by:

- Written guidelines

- Workshop or seminar presentation with overheads, slides or audio visuals

- Repetition of new ideas by other team members

- Key team members meeting with client and family

- Formation of a support group

Practice of new skills with an occupational therapist may include:

- Meal purchasing with assistance

- Meal preparation rehearsal in a therapeutic kitchen

- Immediate feedback on performance

- Assisting clients to understand and adapt to new physical and cognitive behaviour

3.2 PROVIDE NUTRIENT SOURCES

We will consider only the oral intake of foods and/or supplements and factors that may affect purchasing, preparing and presenting meals to the client.

Purchasing involves consideration of:

- Availability from supplier

- Cost of items

- Anticipated usage

- Minimum volume that must be purchased

- Transport to and from supplier

- Use of fresh/frozen/canned products

- Converting meal plan into individual food items i.e. shopping list

Preparing involves consideration of:

- Skill level of cook

- Quantity to be produced

- Availability of pre-prepared items

- Time saving kitchen equipment

- Available time for cooking/preparing

- Ability to safely store excess

- Equipment to prepare supplements

Presentation involves consideration of:

- Distraction-free environment

- Attractive appearance of meal i.e. garnish, sauce

- Suitable cutlery and crockery to encourage independence in eating

- Amount of food and frequency of meals

4. EVALUATE PROGRESS

The purpose of evaluation is to improve the effectiveness of intervention strategies in meeting the clients' needs.

4.1 MEASURE CLIENT SATISFACTION

This is often difficult to accurately gauge as it is dependent on verbal and non-verbal feedback to team members. The psychologist can provide valuable assistance in analysing and formulating appropriate responses to client behaviour. Factors that may affect client satisfaction are:

- Degree of cognitive function and level of awareness/insight.

- Resolution of problems or barriers to change.

- Tendency to answer according to family pressure or, for example, to create a favourable impression to please the therapist or others. [20]

- Tendency to underestimate ability due to, for example, ongoing need for attention. [20]

- Client interest which is variable and depends upon the value the client or family places on the information or task.

- Relevance of the information to the client.

- Successful achievement of goals with newly acquired skills.

- Lack of available education.

All the above factors can result in the client being unable or unwilling to demonstrate competence with the objectives of the nutritional care plan. The decision to revise or replan intervention is made in consultation with the client, family and team members..

4.2 MEASURE THE INTAKE FROM NUTRIENT SOURCES

Food intake may be measured either retrospectively with a diet history (see page 79), or prospectively with food intake and fluid balance charts.

Food Intake

Information recorded on a food intake chart should include:

- General description of food and fluid items.

- Amounts offered (education of professional and family caregivers on the serving volumes of eating utensils, cups and food containers will assist in nutrient calculations).

- Times of meals and snacks.

FOOD INTAKE CHART (Ward & Soft)*

Surname | First Names

CONSISTENCY (WARD | SOFT) SERVING SIZE (S | M | L) DAY..DATE........................

FOOD DESCRIPTION	Amount Offered	Amount Eaten	Calculations (Dietitian)
BREAKFAST			
Yoghurt			
Fruit Juice			
Compote of Fruit			
Cereal......................			
Porridge			
Milk			
Sugar			
Bread/Toast			
Butter/Margarine			
Jam/Honey/Vegemite			
Eggs (poached/ scrambled/boiled)			
Cream			
Baked Beans.............			
Pasta			
Other (describe).........			
MORNING TEA			
Tea/Coffee/"Aktavite"			
Biscuits			
Butter/Margarine			
Cheese.....................			
Fruit.........................			
Milk			
Fruit Juice.................			
Supplement Drink......			
LUNCH			
Soup			
Meat/Fish/Chicken			
Sauce/Gravy/			
Salad Dressing			
Potato (boil/mash/ roast/chipped)			
Other Vegetables.......			
Sandwich			
Meat Salad			
Side Salad			
Dessert.....................			
Jelly Juice.................			
Icecream			
Cream			
Fruit (Fresh/Tinned)....			
Cheese and Biscuit....			
Other (describe).........			
....			

FOOD DESCRIPTION	Amount Offered	Amount Eaten	Calculations (Dietitian)
AFTERNOON TEA			
Tea/Coffee/"Aktavite"			
Biscuits/Cake			
Butter/Margarine			
Cheese.....................			
Fruit.........................			
Milk			
Fruit Juice.................			
Supplement Drink.....			
DINNER			
Soup			
Meat/Fish/Chicken			
Sauce/Gravy/			
Salad Dressing			
Potato (boil/mash/ roast/chipped)			
Other Vegetables.......			
Sandwich			
Meat Salad			
Side Salad			
Bread			
Dessert......................			
Fruit (Fresh/Tinned)....			
Jelly Juice.................			
Icecream			
Cream			
Cheese and Biscuits..			
Other (describe).........			
SUPPER			
Tea/Coffee/"Aktavite"			
Biscuits/Cake			
Butter/Margarine			
Cheese.....................			
Fruit.........................			
Milk			
Fruit Juice.................			
Supplement Drink......			
TOTAL			

APPETITE [Poor | Good]

TIME TO EAT MEAL [◀1/2 hr | 1/2 hr ▶]

* FOOD ITEMS WILL VARY DEPENDING ON INSTITUTION MENU

FOOD INTAKE CHART (Minced & Vitamised)*

Surname	First Names

CONSISTENCY (MINCED | VITAMIZED)   SERVING SIZE (S | M | L)   DAY..............................DATE..........................

FOOD DESCRIPTION	Amount Offered	Amount Eaten	Calculations (Dietitian)	FOOD DESCRIPTION	Amount Offered	Amount Eaten	Calculations (Dietitian)
BREAKFAST				**AFTERNOON TEA**			
Yoghurt				Tea/Coffee/"Aktavite"			
Fruit Juice Jelly				Jellied Cake...............			
Compote of Fruit				Fruit.........................			
Cereal........................				Milk			
Porridge				Jelly Juice.................			
Milk				Supplement Drink......			
Sugar				**DINNER**			
Baked Beans.............				Soup			
Pasta........................				Modified Sandwich			
Eggs (scrambled).......				Meat/Fish/Chicken			
Cream				Sauce/Gravy			
Other (describe).........				Pasta........................			
....				Rice..........................			
....				Potato (mashed)			
MORNING TEA				Green Vegetables			
Tea/Coffee/"Aktavite"				Orange/Yellow			
Jellied Cake...............				Vegetables			
Fruit.........................				Custard			
Milk				Mousse			
Jelly Juice.................				Sago			
Supplement Drink......				Fruit.........................			
LUNCH				Jelly Juice.................			
Soup				Icecream			
Modified Sandwich				Cream			
Meat/Fish/Chicken				Sponge Cake			
Sauce/Gravy				Other (describe).........			
Pasta........................				**SUPPER**			
Rice..........................				Tea/Coffee/"Aktavite"			
Potato (mashed)				Jellied Cake...............			
Green Vegetables				Fruit.........................			
Orange/Yellow				Milk			
Vegetables				Jelly Juice.................			
Custard				Supplement Drink......			
Mousse				**TOTAL**			
Sago							
Jelly Juice.................							
Icecream							
Cream							
Fruit.........................							
Sponge Cake							
Other (describe).........							
....				APPETITE [Poor	Good]			
....							
....				TIME TO EAT MEAL [◀1/2 hr	1/2 hr ▶]			

* FOOD ITEMS WILL VARY DEPENDING ON INSTITUTION MENU

- Amount eaten.

- Time taken to eat the meal.

- Any problems encountered, such as aspiration or vomiting.

Fluid Balance

Fluid requirements are approximately 1500 to 2000 ml per day and may be significantly contributed to by the water content of some foods such as jelly, custard, yoghurt, milk, cooked pasta and rice, fruit, vegetables.

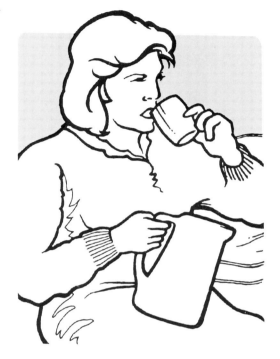

Information recorded on fluid balance charts should include:

Intake -

- Description of the type of fluid.

- Times that fluids were offered.

- The amount of fluid offered.

- Volume of fluid taken by mouth or alternatives such as intravenous or tube feeding.

- Time taken to give fluid volume.

- Total fluid intake after 24 hours.

Output -

- Volume of urine.

- Consistency and amount of fecal output.

- Volume of vomitus or aspirate.

- Time of all fluid output.

4.3 MEASURE THE EFFECT OF NUTRIENT SOURCES

Assessment tools can be selected which are sensitive to changes in conditions requiring intervention. According to the clinical situation and anticipated prognosis, detection of gross changes such as weight and protein status may be followed by more sensitive assessment tools to detect corrigible causes of malnutrition. [21, 22, 23, 24]

DAILY FLUID BALANCE CHART

Surname	First Names	Date

INTAKE					OUTPUT					
Time	By Mouth	ml	Intravenous or Enteral	ml	Vomitus or Aspirate	ml	Feces and Other Drainage (Description)	ml	Urine ml
	....		....		....		....		....
	....		....		....		....		....
	....		....		....		....		....
	....		....		....		....		....
	....		....		....		....		....
	....		....		....		....		....
	....		....		....		....		....
	....		....		....		....		....
	....		....		....		....		....
	....		....		....		....		....
	....		....		....		....		....
	....		....		....		....		....
	....		....		....		....		....
	....		....		....		....		....
	....		....		....		....		....
	....		....		....		....		....
	....		....		....		....		....
	....		....		....		....		....
	....		....		....		....		....
	....		....		....		....		....
	....		....		....		....		....
	....		....		....		....		....
	Sub Total		Sub Total		Sub Total		Sub Total		
	Grand Total						Grand Total		

(Not including Insensible Loss)

(At 2400 hours total input and output to be recorded in the Fluid Balance Summary)

Plus Balance..

Anthropometrics

This involves measuring physical parameters of nutrition such as height, weight, muscle mass, fat stores and either comparing to acceptable standards, or making subsequent comparisons to assess an individual's progress.

Note that most standards available are for 'healthy' people and the clinician's judgement must be used in interpreting results. In evaluating gross measurements such as weight, muscle mass and fat stores, it is best and simplest to look at the person and form a judgement which is necessarily subjective, rather than be bound by healthy standards. In the long term care setting, standards for healthy weight, muscle mass and fat stores are simply not available.

Weight -

It is important where possible to record weight on a regular basis, usually the same day and time each week, but care should be taken in interpreting results. Dehydration and fluid retention may mask weight changes. Rate of weight change is associated with energy intake and results in alterations to protein and fat stores. An increase of 1.0kg/week requires 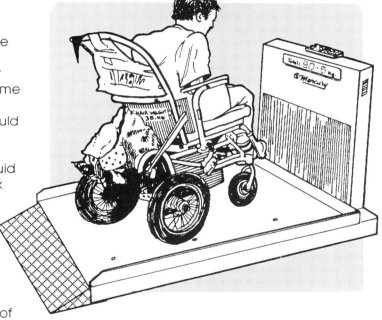 4286 K Joules (1000 K calories) per day above requirements or vice versa. Where muscles have atrophied due to reduced use or catabolic states a goal or ideal weight can be difficult to determine and should be based on the usual weight and extent of muscle and fat loss and anticipated extent of repletion.

Muscle Mass -

Skeletal or somatic muscle mass comprises approximately two thirds of total body protein and can be estimated by several techniques.

The simplest method is to visually compare current physique to pre-trauma photographs of client, or interview family about the client's usual build.

CLIENT CENTRED NUTRITION

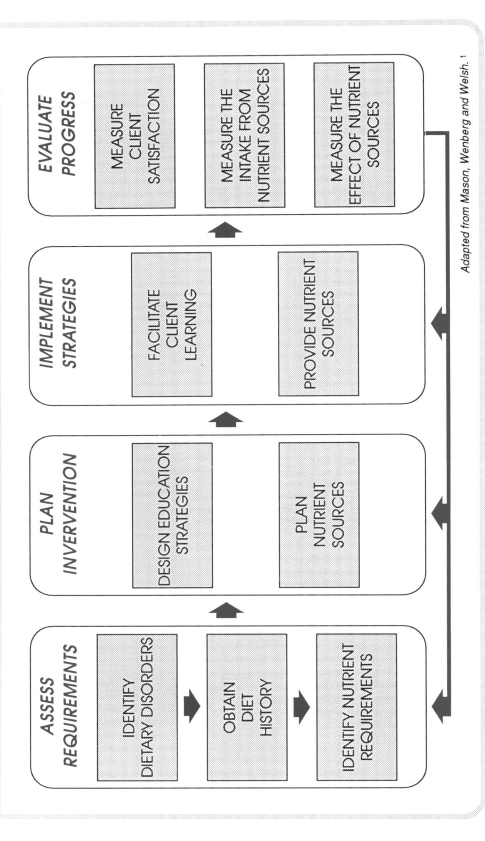

ASSESS REQUIREMENTS
- IDENTIFY DIETARY DISORDERS
- OBTAIN DIET HISTORY
- IDENTIFY NUTRIENT REQUIREMENTS

PLAN INVERVENTION
- DESIGN EDUCATION STRATEGIES
- PLAN NUTRIENT SOURCES

IMPLEMENT STRATEGIES
- FACILITATE CLIENT LEARNING
- PROVIDE NUTRIENT SOURCES

EVALUATE PROGRESS
- MEASURE CLIENT SATISFACTION
- MEASURE THE INTAKE FROM NUTRIENT SOURCES
- MEASURE THE EFFECT OF NUTRIENT SOURCES

Adapted from Mason, Wenberg and Welsh. [1]

An objective method is to estimate muscle mass from measuring mid-arm muscle circumference (MAMC), however there is the potential for user error in untrained clinicians and it is generally only used in clinical trials.

Fat Stores -

Fat is stored predominantly under the skin and rapid depletion of these stores results in loose skin that may be easily grasped between two fingers. An objective method is to estimate subcutaneous fat stores by measuring skin fold thickness, using calipers, however there is the potential for user error in untrained clinicians and it is generally only used in clinical trials.

Biochemistry

Routine multiple biochemical analysis in stable medical conditions is usually carried out six-monthly. Specific biochemical investigations are only conducted to elucidate possible causes of malnutrition or in unstable medical conditions.

ALTERNATIVE FEEDING

For most people with severe swallowing difficulties or altered levels of consciousness, oral intake is limited in some way and may be totally discontinued for safety reasons. Where this occurs the daily intake of foods and fluids, including medications, must be provided by an alternative means. Provision of nutrients by an alternate route requires that certain normal physiological processes involved in eating are by-passed. The type of alternative feeding used will be dependent upon the functional ability available for digesting and absorbing nutrients. For the purposes of this manual, alternative feeding will be considered as either parenteral or tube feeding.

1. PARENTERAL NUTRITION

This term describes any route of nutrient administration other than via the gastro-intestinal tract, although the intravenous is the most commonly used. This method of feeding is generally only used where the gastro-intestinal tract is not functioning.

2. TUBE FEEDING

Where there is a functioning gastro-intestinal tract, tube feeding is the preferred method of providing alternative nutrition. [25, 26]

We have found the following procedures and guidelines to be useful and effective in transitional feeding and general tube feed management.

2.1 FORMULA

Consideration should be given to: [27]

- The functioning level of the digestive and absorptive capacity of the gastro-intestinal tract.

- Relevant pathology, such as renal failure or raised intracranial pressure.

- The metabolic state of the client, whether catabolic or hypermetabolic.

- The effect of previous or present therapy on tolerance and utilisation of the formula.

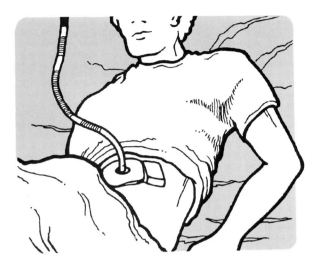

- The client's current nutritional status and possible elevated and/or restricted nutrient requirements.

- The effect of formula on electrolyte balance and specific requirements.

- The presence of underlying metabolic disorders or organ failures that will affect nutrient or fluid requirements.

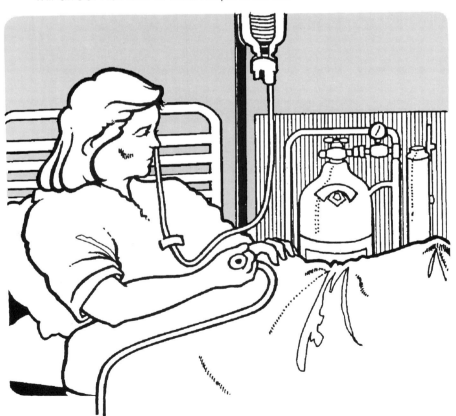

- With a functioning gastro-intestinal tract preferably select a polymeric, iso-osmolar formulae whether feeding into the stomach or small intestine.

- Long term tube feeds require supplementation with trace elements, available in selected formulae.

2.2 TUBE LOCATION

The tip of the tube may be placed either in the stomach or small intestine, and the following factors should be considered: [28]

Stomach

+ Readily tolerates a variety of formulae with varying protein, fat and carbohydrate content.

+ Accepts high osmotic loads with minimal cramping, distension, vomiting, diarrhea, or fluid and electrolyte shifts.

+ Large reservoir capacity for accepting bolus feedings.

+ Tube tip is easily positioned.

- Increased risk of aspiration of refluxed stomach contents.

Small Intestine

+ Reduced risk of aspiration, especially with altered gag, swallow and cough reflexes, lower esophageal sphincter function and gastro-paresis or delayed gastric emptying.

- Care must be taken to avoid the dumping syndrome by initially giving continuous iso-osmolar formulae. [6]

- Accidental retrograde dislodgement of the tube into the stomach, with resultant vomiting, may increase the risk of aspiration.

2.3 ADMINISTRATION

Consideration should be given to the suitability of continuous versus intermittent feeding:

Continuous

+ Preferable when delivering nutrients to the small intestine, which has a poor tolerance to sudden changes in rates of administration and bolus feeds. [29]

+ Reduced gastric residue and improved tolerance where gastric stasis is a concern.

+ Decreased risk of abdominal distension and reflux aspiration of refluxed stomach contents. [30]

- + Possibly greater nutrient delivery, requiring less time to meet nutritional goals. [31]

- - The client must remain attached to the delivery apparatus.

- - Significantly more time-consuming when drip infusion rather than a pump is used.

Intermittent

- + More closely resembles a normal eating pattern. [32]

- + Relatively inexpensive and more convenient in allowing the client to be more mobile.

- + Provides more rest for the gastro-intestinal tract.

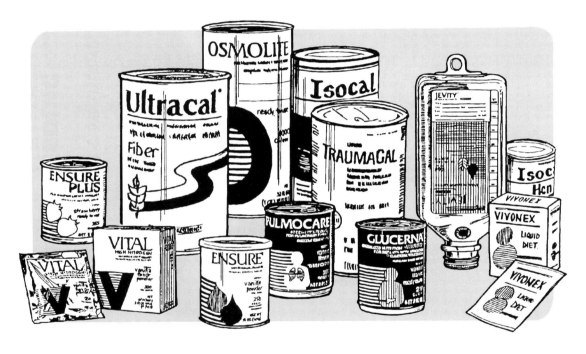

- + Allows for safer pulmonary therapy, such as percussion and drainage on an empty stomach. [33]

- + Reduces the risk of accidental aspiration by an agitated client displacing the tube. [33]

- + May improve stimulation of digestion by greater gastric distension. [28]

- - Excessive distension may retard gastric emptying and increase the risk of aspiration in those prone to reflux. [30, 34]

- - Poorly tolerated when delivered to the small intestine. [29]

2.4 TUBES

In choosing the appropriate feeding tube, consideration should be given to: [35]

- The appropriateness of inserting either a nasal tube or a percutaneous endoscopic gastrostomy (PEG), however the PEG does have the advantages of being cosmetically more appealing, more difficult to accidentally remove and more comfortable.

- The decision to change someone from a nasal tube to a PEG should be based on:
  - * client/family requests,
  - * if a nasogastric tube is constantly needing to be replaced,
  - * if inserting a nasogastric tube is traumatic,
  - * in anticipation of long term tube feeding,
  - * for aesthetic reasons,
  - * or if there is a need for regular tube replacement.

- Length of the tube relative to the desired placement of the tip, i.e. pre or post pylorically.

- Gauge of the tube best suited to any physical restrictions, such as nasal or esophageal restriction, viscosity of the selected formula, mucosal irritation etc.

- General factors affecting the client, such as the presence of a tracheostomy tube, the degree of co-operation or agitation and risk of rejection and withdrawal, and depth of coma.

- Whether a pump is required to ensure a constant flow.

- The anticipated duration of tube feeding.

- Cost and availability of replacement tubes.

2.5 IMPLEMENTATION

Training and procedures are developed to assist nursing staff, clients and family in implementing the tube feeding regime. The following checklist may be helpful: [36]

- ✓ Inservice education on correct use, assembly and maintenance of equipment by relevant company representatives.

- ✓ Aspirate stomach contents prior to the commencement of each feed using a syringe, measure volume and return to stomach. Delay commencement of the next feed if the aspirate volume exceeds 150mls when intermittently feeding. [28] If continuously feeding, aspirate t.d.s. (three times daily). The volume aspirated should not exceed the total feeds given over the last two hours.

✓ Ensure correct formula preparation from powder. Open tin of formula, and store according to instructions on tin to avoid contamination.

✓ Fill formula container at eye level for accurate quantity.

✓ Clear air bubbles from giving set.

✓ Always flush tubing with water from a syringe (water under pressure) before and after giving formula, medication or other strained liquids.

✓ Use correct cleaning procedure if re-using equipment, such as: [37]

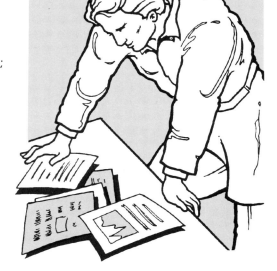

* remove air filter from formula container to ensure it remains dry;
* remove proteinaceous or organic material from container with bottle brush;
* flush tubing with syringe (joined with small piece of wider bore plastic tubing) of warm water,'milton solution', then water;
* immerse container in warm soapy water;
* soak for 1 hour in diluted'milton solution' before using.

✓ Clear blocked tubes as soon as possible by : [38]

* flushing with water using a syringe;
* remove remaining liquid by aspirating with a syringe then flush with a pancreatic enzyme (viokase);
* replace tube.

✓ Ensure correct medication administration by: [36]

* giving medication separately from formulae;
* flushing tube with water before and after medication;
* using liquid medication where possible, or finely crushed tablets with 10-15 ml water;
* giving liquid medication first, then those that need to be diluted; thick medications should be given last.

✓ Replace tubes accidentally removed as soon as possible. Where there is a stoma (percutaneous gastrostomies) then the stoma should be maintained with non-toxic tubing as it may close over within 1 hour. Trained staff should be called in for these tasks.

2.6 MONITORING

The following check list may be helpful to nursing staff and caregivers:

✓ Confirm correct placement by aspiration of gastric contents and testing for acidity. If no gastric aspirate can be obtained, an x-ray should be considered to confirm the position of the tip of the tube.

✓ Elevate head and trunk of the client to the correct feeding position (30°- 45°), before feeding.

✓ Documentation:

* Client's name and identifier number.
* Formula (Name).
* Volume (Total/24 hr.).
* Rate of feeding (mls per hour).
* Duration of feeding/Number of feeds.
* Additional water (ml/hr or flush).

✓ Aspirate at regular intervals to ensure adequate absorption of the feed and correct positioning of the tube.

✓ Discard feed if it has been left open or has been at room temperature for too long (8 hours is the usual maximum).
There is a significant risk of bacterial growth, and staphylococcal enteritis or toxaemia acquired in this way can be fatal. [39]

✓ Record intake and output over 24 hours. Chart volume of water separately.

✓ Record daily number of bowel movements, presence of diarrhea or constipation and stool consistency.

✓ Weigh client once per week.

✓ Correct cleaning procedure for giving set and feeding container at completion of feed and changed on a regular basis. [37]

✓ Dietitian to monitor nutritional status of client.

2.7 COMPLICATIONS

Complications associated with tube feeding can be divided into three main categories: gastrointestinal, mechanical and metabolic. [40]

Care must be taken to document all therapy (medication, medical condition, tube feeds) occurring prior to and during any episodes of complication to help to isolate possible causes.

The following enteral feeding symptoms and considerations may be helpful:

Gastrointestinal Symptoms [40, 41, 42]

- Nausea/Cramping/Flatulence

  Consider:
  * *Cold formula*
  * *Air in feedline*
  * *Lactose/Sucrose intolerance*

- Vomiting

  Consider:
  * *Client positioning 35° - 45°*
  * *Pressure on stomach*
  * *Viral infection*
  * *Medication*
  * *Feed given too rapidly*
  * *Excessive volume of feed*
  * *Esophageal valve incompetence*

- Diarrhea

  Consider:
  * *Fat malabsorption*
  * *Lactose/Sucrose intolerance*
  * *Cold formula*
  * *Medications*
  * *Viral infection in client*
  * *Bacterial contamination of feed*
  * *Fibre content of formula*
  * *Hypoalbuminemia*

- Constipation

  Consider:
  * *Epsom salts*
  * *Lactulose*
  * *Suppositories*
  * *Water intake*
  * *Fibre in formula*

- Steatorrhea

  Consider:
  * *Fat malabsorption*

- Inadequate gastric emptying/ Abdominal distension

  Consider:
  * *Low fat formula*
  * *Iso-osmolar formulae*
  * *Medications*
  * *Continuous delivery*
  * *Client position 35° - 45°*
  * *Volume of feed*
  * *Gastric motitility stimulant, i.e. 'maxolon'*
  * *Position client right side down*
  * *Cool feed down slightly*
  * *Medical investigation*

- Malabsorption

  Consider:
  * *Elemental formulae*

- Gastrointestinal bleeding

  Consider:
  * *Gastric ulcer*

Mechanical Problems [40, 43]

- Feeding tube blockage.

  Consider:
  * *Flushing tube with water after each feed or on a regular basis.*
  * *Medication given down tube adhering to sides of the tube. Note some drugs are incompatible with feeding formulae.*
  * *Tube replacement.*

- Aspiration pneumonia (caused by reflux aspiration of gastric contents or inhalation of secretions).

  Consider:
  * *The correct positioning of the tube tip.*
  * *The correct positioning of the person (preferably 30° - 45° from supine).*
  * *Positioning of the tip of the tube beyond the pylorus to reduce the risk of aspiration.*
  * *Use of polymeric, iso-osmolar formulae administered continuously.*

- Mucosal erosions.

  Consider:
  * *Appropriateness of the diameter or gauge of the tube.*

- Dislocation of feeding tube.

  Consider:
  * *Appropriateness of feeding tube selection*

Metabolic Symptoms [40, 41]

- Serum electrolyte abnormalities.

  Consider:
  * *Formula solute loading*
  * *Supplement formula*

- Macro or micro nutrient deficiencies.

  Consider:
  * *Formulae with trace elements*
  * *Supplement formula*

- Fluid imbalances.

  Consider:
  * *Renal or hepatic disorders.*
  * *Fluid overload.*

- Glucose intolerance.

  Consider:
  * *Insulin*
  * *Carbohydrate content of the formula.*

- Hyperosmotic coma or organ system failure leading to malassimilation of/or the inability to metabolise specific nutrients.

  Consider:
  * *Modifications to the extent of predigestion and proportion of nutrients in the formula.*

TUBE FEEDING

FORMULA	LOCATION	ADMINISTRATION	TUBE	IMPLEMENTATION	MONITORING	COMPLICATIONS
• digestion/ absorption	• stomach	• continuous	• length	• education	• placement	• gastrointestinal
• fluid restrictions	• small intestine	• intermittent	• gauge	• aspiration	• positioning	• mechanical
• medical therapy			• neuro-logical condition of person	• formulae contamination	• documentation	• metabolic
• metabolism			• pumps	• accuracy	• contamination	
• nutrient require-ments			• duration	• air bubbles	• fluid balance	
• electrolytes			• costs	• water flush	• bowels charts	
• metabolic disorders				• cleaning tubes	• weight	
				• blocked tubes	• equipment	
				• medication	• dietitian	
				• dislodgement		

CHAPTER 4 REFERENCES
Nutrition & Alternative Feeding

1.   Mason M, Wenberg BG, Welsh PK. *Process for nutritional counselling.* In: *The dynamics of clinical dietetics.* 2nd ed. New York:Wiley and Sons, 1982:161-260.
2.   Fleisher D, Sheth N, Kou JH. *Phenytoin interaction with enteral feedings administered through nasogastric tubes.* J Parent Ent Nutr 1990; 14(5):513-6.
3.   Thomas J ed. *Prescription products guide 1991.* Australia, 20th ed: Australian Pharmaceutical Publishing Company Ltd. 1781 pp.
4.   Valli C, Schulthess HK, Asper R, Escher F, Hacki WH. *Interaction of nutrients with antacids: a complication during enteral tube feeding.* Lancet 1986; 1:747-8.
5.   Greene HL. *Anatomy and physiology of the intestinal tract.* In: Greene HL, (ed). *Enteral Nutrition:* mead johnson symposium series no. 2. Amsterdam: Exerpta Medica 1984: 1-16.
6.   Wilson PC. *Disorders which adversely affect intestinal function.* In: Greene H.L., (ed). *Enteral Nutrition:* mead johnson symposium series no. 2. Amsterdam: Exerpta Medica, 1984: 26-43.
7.   Bivins BA, Twyman DL, Young AB. *Failure of non protein calories to mediate protein conservation in brain-injured patients.* J of Trauma 1986; 26: 980-6.
8.   Clifton GL, Robertson CS, Grossman RG, Hodge S, Foltz R, Garza C. *The metabolic response to severe head injury.* J Neurosurg 1984; 60: 687-96.
9.   Clifton GL, Robertson CS, Choi SC. *Assessment of nutritional requirements of head-injured patients.* J Neurosurg 1986; 64: 895-901.
10. *Disturbances in water and electrolyte balance and in hydrogen ion concentration.* In: Macleod J, (ed). *Davidson's principles and practice of medicine.* Great Britain: Pitman Press, 1984: 88-103.
11. Dreosti IE. *Recommended dietary intake for protein in Australia.* J Nutr Diet 1989; 46(4):82-92.
12. National Health and Medical Research Council ed. *Dietary allowances for use in Australia.* Canberra: Australian Government Publishing Service, 1984: 16-7.
13. Warwick PM. *Predicting food energy requirements from estimates of energy expenditure.* Aust J Nutr Diet 1989; 46:3-28.
14. Thomas B, ed. *Therapeutic dietetics for disease states.* In: *Manual of dietetic practice.* London: Blackwell Scientific Publications, 1988: 333-534.
15. Bandler R, Grinder J. *The structure of magic.* In: *The structure of magic.* California: Science and Behaviour Books, Inc., 1975: 39-56.
16. Baghurst KI, Hertzler AA, Record SJ, Spurr C. *The development of a simple dietary assessment and education tool for use by individuals and nutrition educators.* J Nutr Edn: "in press".
17. Backhouse JM, Martin J. *Good looking easy swallowing: creative catering for modified texture diets.* Adelaide: Julia Farr Centre Foundation: "in press".
18. Committee on Diet and Health, Food and Nutrition Board, Commission on Life Sciences, National Research Council, eds. *Diet and health: implications for reducing chronic disease risk.* Washington, D.C.: National Academy Press, 1989: 259-71.
19. Committee on Diet and Health, Food and Nutrition Board, Commission on Life Sciences, National Research Council, eds. *Diet and Health: implications for reducing chronic disease risk.* Washington, D.C.: National Academy Press, 1989: 159-258.
20. Silverman I, Shulman AD. *A conceptual model of art; fact in attitude change studies.* Sociometry, 1974; 97-107
21. Taylor KB, Anthony LE. *Assessment of nutritional status.* In: Ferrara AR, Boynton SD, (eds). *Clinical Nutrition.* New York: McGraw-Hill, 1983: 9-34.

22. Clark DG, Sigman R. *Short communication: a simple form for nutritional evaluation.* J. Parent Ent Nutr 1978; 2: 567-8.
23. Blackburn GL, Bistrian BR, Maini BS, *Nutritional and metabolic assessment of the hospitalised patient.* J. Parent Ent Nutr 1977; 11-23.
24. Jensen TG, Englert DM, Dudrich SJ. *Guidelines for interpreting nutritional assessment data.* In: *Nutritional assessment: a manual for practitioners.* Connecticut: Prentice Hall, 1983: 149-206.
25. McArdle AH, Palmason C, Morency I, Brown RA. *A rationale for enteral feeding as the preferable route for hyperalimentation.* Surgery 1981; 90: 616-23.
26. Turner VW. *Nutritional considerations in the patient with disabling brain disease.* Neurosurg 1985 ; 16: 707-13.
27. Gormican A, Liddy E. *Nasogastric tube feedings: practical considerations in prescription and evaluation.* Postgrad Med 1973; 53: 71-6.
28. Rombeau JL. *Methods of enteral feeding.* In: Green HL, (ed). *Enteral Nutrition: Mead Johnson symposium series no. 2.* Amsterdam: Exerpta Medica, 1984: 44-65.
29. Rombeau JL, Barot LR. *Enteral nutrition therapy.* Surg Clin North Am 1981; 61: 605-20.
30. Orr G, Wade J, Bothe A, Blackburn G. *Alternatives to total parenteral nutrition in the critically ill patient.* Crit Care Med 1980; 8: 29-33.
31. Hieberg JM, Brown A, Anderson RG, Halfacre S, Rodeheaver GT, Edlich RF. *Comparison of continuous versus intermittent tube feedings in adult burn patients.* J Parent Ent Nutr 1981 ; 5 : 73-5.
32. Perkins MR. *Bolus enteral feeding.* J Food Nutr 1985; 42 :195-6.
33. Kolan MJ, Hickish SM. *A comparison of continuous and intermittent enteral nutrition in NICU patients.* J Neurosci Nursing 1986 ; 18: 333-7.
34. Heitkemper ME, Martin DL, Hansen BL, Hanson R, Vanderburg V. *Rate and volume of intermittent enteral feeding.* J Parent Ent Nutr 1981; 5 :125-9.
35. Gordon AM. *Enteral nutrition support : guidelines for feeding tube selection and placement.* Post Grad Med 1981; 70 :155-62.
36. Nursing Procedures Committee, *Gastrostomy: feeding, tube care, wound care and medication administration.* In: Julia Farr Centre procedure manual. Adelaide: Julia Farr Centre, 1991 :E 14.1.
37. Nursing Procedures Committee. *Cleansing of enteric feeding equipment using milton anti-bacterial solution.* In: Julia Farr Centre procedure manual. Adelaide: Julia Farr Centre, 1991 :E 12.2.
38. Marcuard SP, Stegel KS. *Unclogging feeding tubes with pancreatic enzyme.* J Parent Ent Nutr 1990; 14 :198-9.
39. Cameron A, ed. *Guidelines for preventing contamination of enteral feedings.* In: Cameron A, Redfern DE, eds. Report of the Ross workshop on contamination of enteral feeding products during clinical usage. Columbus, Ohio: Ross Laboratories, 1983: 40-2.
40. Cataldi-Betcher EL, Seltzer MH, Slocum BA, Jones KW. *Complications occurring during enteral nutrition support: a prospective study.* J Parent Ent Nutr 1983; 7: 546-52.
41. Silk DBA. *Towards the optimization of enteral nutrition.* Clin Nutr 1987; 6: 61-74.
42. Silk DBA. *Fibre and enteral nutrition.* Gut 1989; 30: 246-64.
43. Kleibeuker J. H., Boersma-Van W. *Acute effects of continuous nasogastric tube feeding on gastric function: comparison of a polymeric and a nonpolymeric formula.* J Parent Ent Nutr 1991; 15 : 80-4.

ASPIRATION, CHOKING AND EMERGENCY PROCEDURES

It is the responsibility of every healthcare worker to be familiar and confident with performing emergency procedures on clients who present with swallowing dysfunction. Too often the client is put 'at risk' when certain foods and fluids are given haphazardly in an attempt to alleviate swallowing problems.

Before beginning swallowing, eating, or feeding management, staff and family carers should be familiar with the important relationship between breathing and swallowing, and what to do should something 'go wrong'.

1.RESPIRATORY SYSTEM - AN OVERVIEW

1.1 WHAT MAKES UP THE RESPIRATORY SYSTEM? [2,3]

Nose - Air passes through the nasal passages and dust and other particles are removed. The air on inspiration is warmed and moisture added.

Mouth - Adds to that function of the nose by providing humidity and warmth.

Throat (Pharynx) - Is the physical space that air passes through on its way from the mouth/nose down to the voice box (larynx).

Voice Box (Larynx) - Inside the voice box, at the level of the Adam's Apple, are the vocal cords and flap-like epiglottis. During swallowing both of these act to prevent food and fluid from entering the airway.

Windpipe (Trachea) - Is the large airpipe made of cartilagenous rings that divides into the bronchi, which in turn provide the route for oxygen and carbon dioxide exchange at the level of the alveoli in the lungs.

Diaphragm - Is the large dome-shaped muscle directly under the lungs. Movement of the diaphragm causes air to be drawn in through the nose and mouth, down through the larynx and trachea, finally reaching the alveoli in the lungs (inspiration).

1.2 WHAT HAPPENS WHEN WE BREATHE? [2,3,10]

Breathing is the act by which we obtain oxygen (inspiration), and remove carbon dioxide (expiration) from the blood and lungs. This process is controlled by the action of the vagus nerve and is mediated in the medulla oblongata.

Although breathing is largely involuntary, it involves the muscular activity of the diaphragm (70% of the work) and intercostal muscles between the ribs.

THE RESPIRATORY SYSTEM

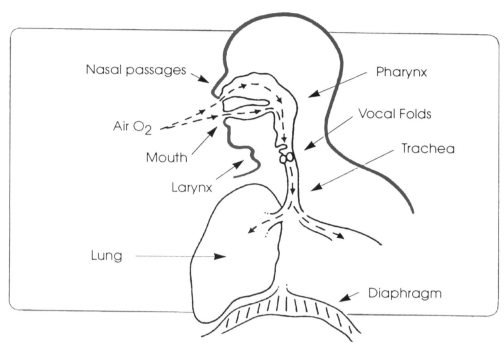

When a person 'breathes in' the diaphragm moves down which causes a partial vacuum and air rushes into the lungs. When a person 'breathes out' the diaphragm is relaxed and returns to its starting position; this pushes air, with excess carbon dioxide, out of the lungs. The intercostal muscles work in conjunction with the diaphragm, changing lateral excursion of the abdominal wall, and thus allowing for sideways expansion of the lungs on inspiration.

1.3 HOW DOES THE RESPIRATORY SYSTEM PROTECT ITSELF? [2,3,9,11]

The respiratory system has various ways of protecting itself from foreign and potentially harmful material, i.e.:

Nose and Mouth -	filter dust and other particles.
Sneeze -	is a reflex which helps clear the nasal passages.
Cough -	is a reflex triggered at the level of the vocal cords to forcefully expel irritating substances and mucous.
Cilia -	are located in the bronchial tree and cleanse the lung of foreign particles by continually moving a thin layer of mucous toward the mouth.
Mucous -	is produced by the lungs as a cleaning agent for the respiratory system. We normally produce ¼ - ½ cup per day.

2. ASSESSMENT OF THE RESPIRATORY SYSTEM[1,3]

The physiotherapist is responsible for assessing respiratory status.

Auscultation- abnormal breath sounds may be indicative of early changes in respiratory status. e.g. distribution of aeration, congestive sounds.

Pulmonary Function Testing - provides objective assessment of vital capacity, expiratory and inspiratory pressure.

Arterial blood gases - can measure level and effectiveness of gas exchange.

Chest X-ray - may reveal areas of consolidation.

Results obtained are discussed with the team to interpret their likely impact on the swallowing process.

It must be stressed that breathing and swallowing are highly synchronised. The act of swallowing is characterised by; momentary cessation of breathing (airway protection)... followed by oral mastication and swallow reflex which initiate the swallowing phase... and on completion of the swallow, inspiration is resumed.

In a normal person swallowing and breathing cannot occur simultaneously.

2.1 TRACHEOSTOMY AND SWALLOWING.

Assessment of the effectiveness of respiration and swallowing in a client with tracheostomy will require knowledge of the type of tube in situ, and the procedure for conducting a methylene blue test.

TRACHEOSTOMY TUBES

1. *Cuffless*

- Bypasses upper airway obstructions.

- Maintains safe ventilation.

- Allows removal of secretions by suction.

- Used when assisted ventilation is no longer required and the risk of aspiration is considered to be no longer a problem.

2. *Cuffless fenestrated*

- Allows a client with a long term tracheostomy increasingly to rely on upper airway breathing.

- Phonation (making sound) is possible.

- Decannulation plug (DCP) can be inserted into the lumen of the outer cannula to direct breathing through the upper air passages.

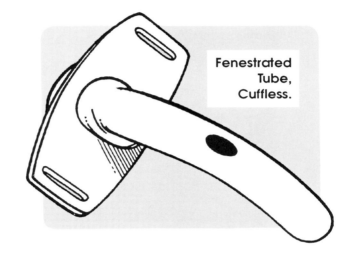

Fenestrated Tube, Cuffless.

3. *Low-pressure cuffed*

- Double airway design permits maintenance of patent airway without removing the entire tube.

- The cylindrical, high volume, low pressure cuff provides an effective seal with minimum pressure.

- A twist-lock connector can be attached to anesthesia and ventilating equipment.

METHYLENE BLUE TEST

The methylene blue procedure provides objective information on the likelihood of regurgitation of gastric contents or aspiration of oral intake.[1]

Warning:
Methylene blue will temporarily stain the teeth and mouth if it is given undiluted. Excessive amounts may be toxic.

Adequate contrast is provided by 0.5ml in 30ml of water.

Procedure

1. With the cuff inflated apply oro-pharyngeal suction above the cuff and endotracheal suction to remove secretions below the cuff.

2. A swallowing assessment can be

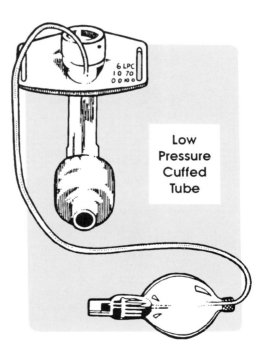

Low Pressure Cuffed Tube

successfully undertaken with the cuff either inflated or deflated.

2.1 *Inflated Cuff*

Cuff inflation should be maintained if the client has a high risk of aspiration. Occasionally the cuff may irritate the trachea or restrict laryngeal elevation.

The test is evaluated by applying oropharyngeal and endotracheal suction.

2.2 *Deflated Cuff*

Cuff deflation may inadvertently place the client at risk of direct aspiration. When the cuff is deflated the tracheostomy tube is less likely to interfere with swallowing. A sputum gutter container may be attached to the catheter for direct collection of residue.

The test is evaluated by applying endotracheal suction.

3. Explain the procedure to the client and bystanders.

4. Administer a small amount (5 - 10 ml) of dye solution orally as a sip, with a syringe or as a jelly, and ask the client to hold the substance in the mouth.

5. Direct the client to swallow purposefully. You may need to demonstrate this. Any evidence of direct aspiration is noted, and described as coughing before, during or after the swallow.

6. After thirty seconds to a minute apply suction.

7. Analyse the material sucked out:

   • *Positive*: any evidence of blue dye stain suggests possible aspiration.

   • *Negative*: if there is no blue dye detected, aspiration is unlikely.

8. This procedure should be done at least three times at different times and on consecutive days to ensure that the results are valid and reliable.

3. ASPIRATION AND CHOKING

Aspiration and choking are evidence of a respiratory system in difficulty. In the client with acquired neurological dysfunction this may be due to any one or a combination of -

   • swallowing difficulties of bulbar origin resulting in inco-ordination of swallowing musculature and ineffective glottic closure. [2,10]

ASPIRATION
SYSTEM PROTECTING ITSELF

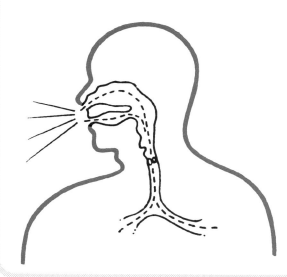

- gagging
- sneezing
- reflexive coughing
- forced expiration

Aspiration is when food, fluid or mucous enters the airway *without total occlusion*. Although uncomfortable and distressing, the client is able to protect the airway without assistance.

CHOKING
SYSTEM NOT EFFECTIVE IN PROTECTING ITSELF

- airway becomes totally obstructed
- breathing ceases (unable to get air down)
- cyanosis develops

Choking is when there is *total occlusion* of the airway by food, fluid or saliva. This is an immediately life-threatening situation, with significant risk of neuronal damage, and early cyanosis with loss of consciousness.

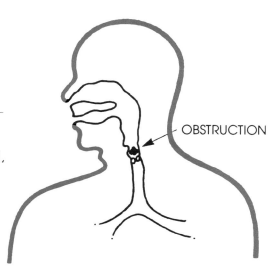

OBSTRUCTION

- weakness of the diaphragm and intercostal muscles resulting in reduced effectiveness of cough reflex. [2,3,10]

- increased secretions, poor management of these and changes in viscosity of mucous.

3.1 ASPIRATION

Aspiration is when food, fluid or saliva enters the airway without total occlusion, usually accompanied by violent coughing, shortness of breath and panic.

Acute Management

Although the individual is uncomfortable and distressed, life is not immediately in danger, and it should be feasible to get enough air down at least partially if not completely to cough up the substance without outside help.

DO NOT HIT ON THE BACK. THE 'HEIMLICH MANOUEVRE' IS NOT RECOMMENDED.
(Australian Resuscitation Council, 1988)[14]

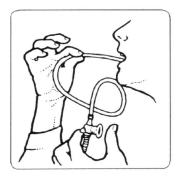 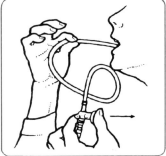 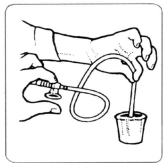

ORAL SUCTIONING TECHNIQUE

Chronic Management

In order to reduce the frequency and degree of chronic aspiration the emphasis should be on prevention and compensation, rather than cure, i.e.

Alterations to minimum standards of feeding -

1. Safest texture and consistency of food, fluid and medication is assessed and recommended on the basis of ease of oral stage management and ability to expectorate, e.g. thickened fluids.

2. Optimum head and body position to promote airway protection.

3. Safe swallowing routine to encourage co-ordination of swallowing and breathing at a conscious level, and promote protection of airway.

4. Optimum environment for meals to reduce distraction: effective cueing and prompting, assistive devices, and post-meal management to reduce the likelihood of aspiration before, during, and after the swallow.

5. Staff management of aspiration including support, counselling, supervision and *oral suctioning* after the event to remove excess residue in the mouth.

Alterations to type of feeding -

1. Gradual transition to alternative feeding as main source of nutrition and hydration will reduce frequency of aspirational episodes.

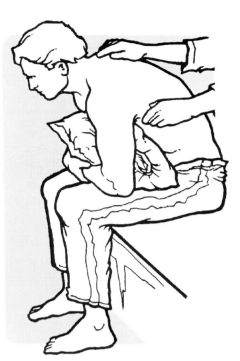

CHEST PHYSIOTHERAPY

2. Change from nasogastric/ gastrostomy site of delivery to jejunostomy to reduce aspiration following reflux or vomiting.

Medical and Surgical intervention [1,3,4,12]

1. Mini-tracheostomy or cuffed tracheostomy tubes allow for control of secretions and maintenance of airway patency. Tracheal suctioning is an efficient method of removing unwanted residue in the lower airway.

2. *Chest physiotherapy* and/or *postural drainage* to the affected area may assist in dislodging build-up of mucous and other secretions.

3. Surgical intervention may be considered in extreme cases, e.g. teflon injection of the vocal cords (to promote firmer closure on adduction),[13], complete laryngectomy, or glottic 'sew-over'.

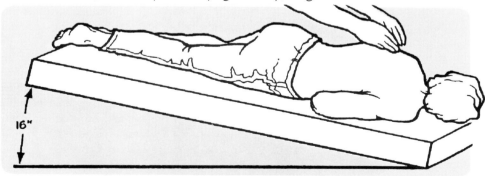

16"

POSTURAL DRAINAGE

3.2 CHOKING

Choking refers to an event where there is total occlusion of the airway by food, fluid or saliva.

This is an immediately life-threatening situation, with significant risk of neuronal damage, and early cyanosis with loss of consciousness.

EMERGENCY TREATMENT

1. *A background of controversy and debate.*

The skills and knowledge of basic life support need to be consistent, easily understood and documented, and regularly reviewed.

Unfortunately in practice there is no one universally-accepted procedure for choking.

Confusion regarding use of the *Heimlich Manoeuvre* vs *chest thrusts* vs *back slaps* may result in life-threatening hesitation and potential mistakes in the event of choking.

Supporters of the Heimlich Manoeuvre suggest that it delivers strong kinetic energy to a foreign body and it always propels the object toward the mouth and away from the lungs.[10]

Day et al [9,10] reported that the effect of backslap energy is to direct the foreign body toward the lungs, rather than away from the lungs. The energy generated was reported as much less than for the Heimlich Manoeuvre.

Critics of the Heimlich Manoeuvre (American and Australian Red Cross) believe that the various abdominal thrust techniques, using forcible pressure over the abdomen, should not be used as they: [14]

- may damage internal organs, especially the liver, spleen and stomach

- may precipitate regurgitation of stomach contents

- would be dangerous in a pregnant woman (or severely debilitated patients)

2. *Treatment of Choice*

Until conclusive scientific evidence in humans can suggest the preferred treatment, emergency procedures must be devised based upon:

(A) Policy

An Institution or workplace procedural statement that has been developed for the management of choking. For example - the following choking procedural Chart has been adapted from the Australian Resuscitation Council Guidelines [14], and the Julia Farr Nursing Procedures Manual. [15]

IF A PERSON IS CHOKING this is an EMERGENCY - DO NOT LEAVE THE PERSON

(1) Call urgently for help.

(2) Remove dentures if they are present.

(3) Use one or two fingers to scoop any food from the back of the throat towards the mouth. Be careful to avoid making the person vomit. Also take care to avoid pushing any food or obstruction further down the throat.

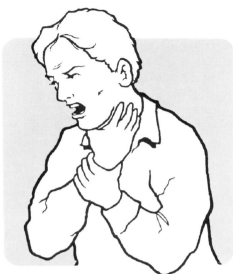

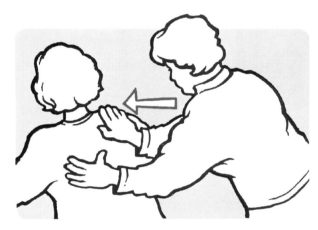

(4) Encourage the person to cough.

(5) If the person is unable to breathe or cough, whilst in an upright (seated) position, slap him/her between the shoulder blades 3 to 4 times using the flat of the hand.

(6) If the person is still unable to breathe or cough, in a sitting position bend him/her at the waist swiftly head towards knees no more than 3 times as this can help to push the obstruction up out of the airway. (Modified Heimlich Manoeuvre)

(7) If the person is still unable to breathe or cough call an ambulance immediately. Lie the person on his side and turn his/her head to be tilted slightly upwards.

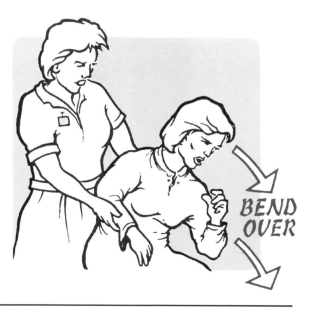

BEND OVER

(B) Individual client characteristics

Although many practitioners report that existing, traditional choking procedures ' don't work on some clients, especially the severely disabled ', we must stress using caution in trying to change these haphazardly. Any modifications to existing procedures must take into account the following factors:

1. The client's assessed problem(s) and the resultant impact on existing choking procedures, e.g. contractures and positioning.

2. That all preventative measures have been trialled and their effectiveness evaluated. (Minimum Standards, see 'Chronic Management of Aspiration', page 120)

3. That any alterations to existing choking procedures be discussed with the medical officer, trialled and evaluated.

All team members, health professionals and family carers, can feel more confident using choking procedures when an educational checklist (see opposite) is reviewed every 3 to 6 months. [9]

EMERGENCY PROCEDURE for CHOKING

EDUCATION CHECKLIST

The following staff and family carers have been
educated regarding choking procedures for

....

(CLIENT)

Name...................................Date	Name.....................................Date ....
Name...................................Date	Name.....................................Date ....
Name...................................Date	Name.....................................Date ....

☐ **1** The client has been taught a pre-determined sign to signal distress during eating or drinking.

☐ **2** Family and staff are familiar with minimum standards of feeding to reduce the likelihood of choking:
- texture and consistency
- head and body positioning
- swallowing routine and assistive devices

☐ **3** Family and staff are familiar with practical emergency procedures for choking.

☐ **4** Key skilled staff are familiar with pharyngeal suction. Need for standby suction has been determined.

☐ **5** All staff and carers are aware of the importance of prompt action including methods of calling for further assistance. i.e. educational leaflets, posters.

☐ **6** Documentation and review processes have been implemented to ensure validity of recommendations.

.... Date.......................
(Signature of Staff Member completing this Form)

CHAPTER 5 REFERENCES
Aspiration, Choking and Emergency Procedures

1. Huff CL. *The Role of Respiratory Therapy in ALS.* In *Amytrophic Lateral Sclerosis: A Teaching Manual for Health Professionals.* Kirkland, Washington: ALS Health Support Services, 1989.
2. Groher ME (ed). *Dysphagia: diagnosis and management.* Boston: Butterworths, 1984.
3. Preston W., Dinohoe K., Ten Eyck LG., Goldblatt D. *Managing Breathing Problems.* In MAL Manual III, *Managing Amyotrophic Lateral Sclerosis*: ALS Association, 1986.
4. Griggs CA., Jones PM., Lee RE. *Videofluoroscopic Investigation of Feeding Disorders of children with Multiple Handicap.* J.Dev.Med Child Neural, 1989: 31:303-8.
5. Feinberg MJ., Ekberg E. *Deglutition after Near Fatal Choking Episode: Radiologic Evaluation.* Radiology, 1990:176:637-640.
6. Titley I., Davidson RN., Turner E., et al. *Fibreoptic bronchoscopy: An assessment of immediate cytological diagnosis using methylene blue stain.* Resp.Med. 1989:83:37-41.
7. Committee on Accident and Poison Prevention. *First Aid for the Choking Child*, 1988. Pediatrics, 1988; 81 No.5:740-742.
8. Sanders HN. *Feeding Dependent Eaters Among Geriatric Patients.* J.Nut.for the Eld, 1990; 9 No.3:69-74.
9. Langston J. *Gasping for Breath.* Nursing Times, 1990; 86 No.33:39-41.
10. Heimlich HJ., Patrick EA. *The Heimlich Manoeuvre.* Postgrad.Med., 1990; 87 No.5:38-53.
11. Logemann J. *Evaluation and treatment of swallowing disorders.* San Diego: College Hill Press Inc., 1983.
12. Hogstel MO., Robinson NB. *Feeding the Frail Elderly.* J of Geron Nurs., 1989; 15 No.3:16-20.
13. Cochrane GM (ed). *The Management of Motor Neurone Disease.* U.K.: Longman Group U.K. Ltd. 1987.
14. Australian Resuscitation Council. *Interim Policy Statement: The management of Choking due to suspected impaction of foreign material in or just above the windpipe.* No. 4.3.6 - March 1988.
15. Nursing Procedures Committee. *Procedure for management of aspiration and choking.* In: Julia Farr Centre Procedure Manual. Adelaide: Julia Farr Centre, 1991: D8.1-6.

6

FACTORS AFFECTING OUTCOME & USEFUL THERAPEUTIC TECHNIQUES

LOCATION AND EXTENT OF THE LESION

The more extensive the brain injury, the poorer the prospects for good functional recovery. The neurological organisation of swallowing is complex and lesions can occur at a number of different levels: [1,2,3]

1. *Sensory (afferent) stimulation of swallow reflex.*

   - Cranial nerves V, IX, X and XII receive sensations from the lips, tongue, palate, pharynx, larynx and joints in the mouth and face.

   - The sensation of taste as registered in the tongue is carried by the VII (anterior two thirds) and IX (posterior one third) nerves. Taste receptors are stimulated by the flavours sweet, sour, salty or bitter. A screening test can be conducted by using a gustometer constructed by adapting a globe fitting for an ophthalmoscope to accept two prongs.

   - Cognitive integration of sight, smell and memory for food preferences occurs in the frontal lobes.

2. *Central organization* and control of the swallow reflex occur in the medulla oblongata, in particular on either side of the midline within the medullary reticular formation.

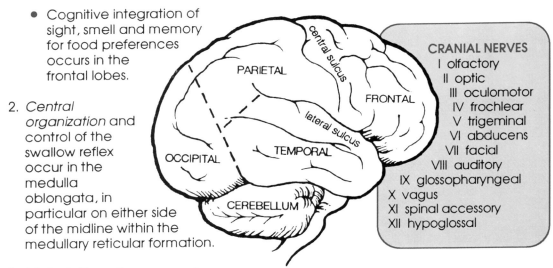

CRANIAL NERVES
I olfactory
II optic
III oculomotor
IV frochlear
V trigeminal
VI abducens
VII facial
VIII auditory
IX glossopharyngeal
X vagus
XI spinal accessory
XII hypoglossal

3. *Motor (efferent) responses* to swallowing involve cranial nerves V, VII, IX and XII. Motor control of salivation from the parotid, sublingual, and submandibular glands is via fibres in the seventh and ninth cranial nerves.

SPONTANEOUS RECOVERY

Spontaneous recovery is expected in most rehabilitation clients, and can take anything from three weeks to three years or more. Perseveration, emotional lability and fluctuating concentration and attention span can contribute to a wide variation in swallowing performance in the initial stages of recovery. [2,3]

MOTIVATION, AWARENESS AND SELF CORRECTION

Clients who are aware of their errors and attempt to correct them have a more favourable prognosis than those who are unable to do so. [2]

INSTABILITY IN MEDICAL AND NUTRITIONAL STATUS

Fluctuations in medical and nutritional status can occur spontaneously, or as a consequence of specific management strategies.[4] For example, myositis ossificans (bone formation in the muscles around joints) often occurs after severe brain injury. If the elbow is involved the fixed deformity can prevent progress in self-feeding until after surgical removal. Intermittent self-limiting complications, such as diarrhea and infections, can interrupt management of the swallowing component of rehabilitation.

TEAM DYNAMICS AND EXPERIENCE

Team dynamics and experience will determine the effectiveness and efficiency of a transitional feeding program. Essential elements in achieving good results are:

- Adequate staffing.

- Team leadership and commitment, including a coherent philosophy.

- Management flexibility to include the family as integral members of the team.

- Readiness by all involved to accept that the personality of skilled feeders is more important than status in a professional hierarchy.

- Clear documentation.

COMPREHENSIVE ASSESSMENT AND PLANNING

Comprehensive assessment and planning are essential in determining the timing of intervention and plans for management. Inadequate team planning can result in unnecessary failure and lack of progress if the initial goals are not clearly achievable.

ETHICAL CONSIDERATIONS

Any form of alternative feeding (enteral and parenteral) should be likened to other medical interventions and not viewed as a routine provision of care and comfort. [5,6]

A difficult situation can arise with a client in the persisting vegetative state, when both family and professional staff are convinced that there is no evidence of residual personality, even many months after the original injury. Commonly, an explicit or implicit clinical policy is adopted of not giving antibiotics for infective complications, but otherwise maintaining care. If a tube becomes blocked or is removed, the question of reinsertion may arise.

If the client is not legally competent or is held to be psychiatrically disturbed, appropriate action is required according to the local legal jurisdiction. In South Australia this would involve approaching the Guardianship Board, perhaps to ask for a Treatment Order.

It is conventional practice to closely involve the family in these issues, but in the final analysis, our ethical obligation is to the client, not to those concerned with the welfare of the client, whether they be family members or professionals seeking to act as advocates. Since a client receiving transitional feeding in such a situation will always be admitted to a hospital nursing home, or hospice under the care of a medical practitioner, the final arbiter must be that person.

These decisions are never easy, may cause much debate amongst members of the team and others concerned for the client, and should be made openly and with full discussion, free from acrimony or rancour.

2. USEFUL THERAPEUTIC PROCEDURES

DESENSITISATION

Clients with severe bilateral frontal brain damage may develop abnormal oral reflexes,[1,3,4] (described in Chapter 3) which must be reduced (desensitised) to allow normal feeding. The following description is intended as a guide, to be modified according to each individual situation.

2.1 *Treatment Program*

- Oro-facial exercises are performed for five minutes, four times daily.

- Only caregivers (family and otherwise) trained and confirmed by the speech pathologist should attempt desensitisation procedures.

- Use the thumbs and index fingers to apply firm pressure to the muscles from the midline to the outside of the face.

SEQUENCE of DESENSITISATION
(all exercises are performed on both sides simultaneously)

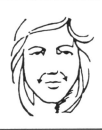 (i) Stroke along upper lip, from the middle downwards towards corners of the mouth. Use firm strokes.

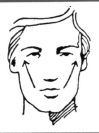 (iii) Stroke across cheeks. Use firm strokes.

(ii) Stroke along lower lip. Start from the middle and work up to the corners of the mouth. Use firm strokes.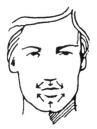

((iv) Use cotton bud probes and lemon glycerine swabs to firmly stroke along outer gums (careful not to touch the teeth).
Right upper gum
Left upper gum
Right lower gum
Left lower gum

- Those involved should take 'universal precautions' (in the sense of infection control procedures), and in particular must wear gloves.

2.2 *Procedure*

- Firmly stroke the muscles of the face.

- Start at the midline and work outwards.

- Stroke each muscle group 10 times.

- Stroke both sides of the face simultaneously.

BRUSHING AND ICING 1,4,5

Before using the following exercises it is essential that a speech pathologist has assessed muscle function and prescribed specific procedures.

- Be prepared to carry out these exercises up to five times per day. If at any time you are in doubt, ask the speech pathologist to review and demonstrate the correct technique.

FACE, LIPS AND TONGUE - *Brushing and Icing*

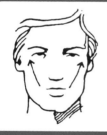 (i) Brush then ice from corner of the mouth to the outside corner of the eye.	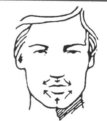 (iv) To encourage lip closure, brush then ice in the direction of the movements i.e. down on the top lip and up on the bottom lip.
(ii) Brush then ice from corner of the mouth to the nostrils. 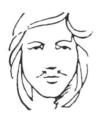	(v) For pursing of the lips, brush then ice around the lips without crossing the midline. Ice the inside lips and between them to encourage closure.
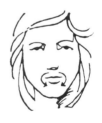 (iii) Brush then ice from over the cheek towards the ear in a zig-zag pattern.	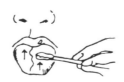 (vi) Brush with iced swab from front to back of tongue without crossing the midline. Ask client to suck on an ice cube, roll it around with the tongue, then spit it out.

- Never cross the midline and work each side separately.

- Begin work on the stronger side of the face, then move to the weaker side.

- Do the brushing exercises first, followed by icing, and then specific muscle exercises or eating.

- After completing brushing and icing exercises the client should be encouraged to make full use of their effect by following the series of exercises below with supervision. Alternatively, eating a meal may be substituted for the exercises below, for the desired muscles will then be exercised.

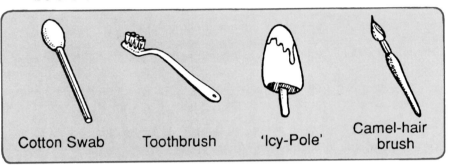

Cotton Swab   Toothbrush   'Icy-Pole'   Camel-hair brush

2.3 *Lip Exercises (5 times each exercise)*

- Make the mouth round to form a whistling shape.

- Move the mouth to a smiling shape.

- Start with a whistle and move to a smile.

- Open the mouth wide, then close.

- Start with a smile, then whistle, then open wide, then close.

2.4 *Tongue Exercises*

- Put the tongue out as far as it will go, and keep it straight if possible.

- Put tongue down to the chin, then up to the nose.

- Move the tongue from one corner of the mouth to the other.

- Move tongue around the teeth.

- Move tongue around the lips.

3. COMA AND OUTCOME SCALES

Refer to **coma and outcome scales** (opposite) used world-wide as guidelines for recovery.

COMA & OUTCOME SCALES — Measures of cognitive status

1. COMA SCALE

Glasgow Coma Scale

Verbal Commands
5 Oriented
4 Disoriented
3 Words
2 Sounds
1 Nil to pain

Best Motor Response
6 Obeys commands
5 Localises pain (purposeful)
4 Flexor withdrawal (semipurposeful)
3 Abnormal flexion (decorticate)
2 Extensor (decerebrate)
1 Nil (flaccid)

Eye Opening
4 Spontaneous
3 To command
2 To pain
1 Nil to pain

Reprint permission obtained from Jennett and Teasdale 1989

2. OUTCOME SCALES

Rancho Los Amigos Outcome Scale (Revised)

1. *No Response*
Patient unresponsive to stimuli.

2. *Generalized Response*
Patient responds inconsistently and nonpurposefully to stimuli. Responses are limited and often delayed.

3. *Localized Response*
Patient reacts specifically but inconsistently to stimuli. Responses are related to type of stimulus presented, such as focusing on an object visually or responding to sounds.

4. *Confused, Agitated*
Patient is extremely agitated and in a high state of confusion. Shows nonpurposeful and aggressive behaviour. Unable to fully co-operate with treatments due to short attention span. Maximal assistance with selfcare skills is needed.

5. *Confused, Inappropriate, Non-agitated*
Patient is alert and can respond to simple commands on a more consistent basis. Highly distractible and needs constant cueing to attend to an activity. Memory is impaired with confusion regarding past and present. The patient can perform selfcare activities with assistance. May wander and needs to be watched carefully.

6. *Confused, Appropriate*
Patient shows goal directed behaviour, but still needs direction from staff. Follows simple tasks consistently and shows carryover for relearned tasks. The patient is more aware of his/her deficits and has increased awareness of self, family and basic needs.

7. *Automatic, Appropriate*
Patient appears oriented in home and hospital and goes through daily routine automatically. Shows carryover for new learning but still requires structure and supervision to ensure safety and good judgement. Able to initiate tasks in which he has an interest.

8. *Purposeful, Appropriate*
Patient is totally alert, oriented, and shows good recall of past and recent events. Independent in the home and community. Shows a decreased ability in certain areas but has learned to compensate.

Reprint permission obtained from the Head Trauma Service of Rancho Los Amigos Medical Center, Downey, C.A., U.S.A.

Santa Clara Valley Disability Rating Scale for Severe Head Trauma: Coma to Community

Primary Level
Patient is very dependent or requires maximal assistance either physically, cognitively perceptually, or in all three areas.

1. *Severe Motor Impairment*
• Severe spasticity
• Abnormal reflexes
• Loss of motor control in any or all four limbs
• Head and trunk control severely impaired
• Dependent in selfcare activities

2. *Severe Impairment of Perceptual Motor Skills*
• Poor/gross visual skills and perceptual motor skills that prevent selfcare or higher functional activities
• Severe motor planning deficits
• Poor visual attentiveness and visual tracking

3. *Decreased Functional Cognition and Behaviour*
• Extremely poor judgement
• Safety, awareness, problem-solving abilities and memory are all severely affected
• Dependent in most functional tasks

Advanced Level
Patient may have cognitive, perceptual, motor and/or behavioural deficits — but these are not significant enough to cause total dependence in activities of daily living.
• Potential to make an adaptive motor response and carryover learning toward achieving a functional goal
• Level of awareness is higher with better ability to control more aspects of the environment and participate in a rehabilitation program
• Therapy is aimed toward functional goals in feeding, dressing and vocation.

Reprint permission obtained from Rappaport and Hall 1988.

CHAPTER 6 REFERENCES
Factors Affecting Outcome & Useful Therapeutic Techniques

1. Roueche JR. *Dysphagia: An assessment and management programme for the adult.* Chicago: Sister Kenny Institute, 1980.
2. Steefel J. *Dysphagia rehabilitation for neurologically impaired adults.* Springfield: Charles C Thomas, 1981.
3. Veis SL, Logemann JA. *The nature of swallowing disorders in CVA patients.* Arch Phys Med Rehabil 1985; 66: 372-375.
4. Kalisky Z, Morrison DP, Meyers CA. *Medical problems encountered during rehabilitation of patients with head injury.* Arch Phys Med Rehabil 1985; 66: 25-29.
5. Padilla GV, Grant M, Wong H, et al. *Subjective distresses of nasogastric tube feeding.* J Parent Enter Nutrit 1979; 3 (2): 53-57.
6. Pavis JF. *When burdens of feeding outweigh benefits.* Hastings Centre Report 1986: 30-32.

INDEX

(Bold Numbers denote Illustration or Chart)